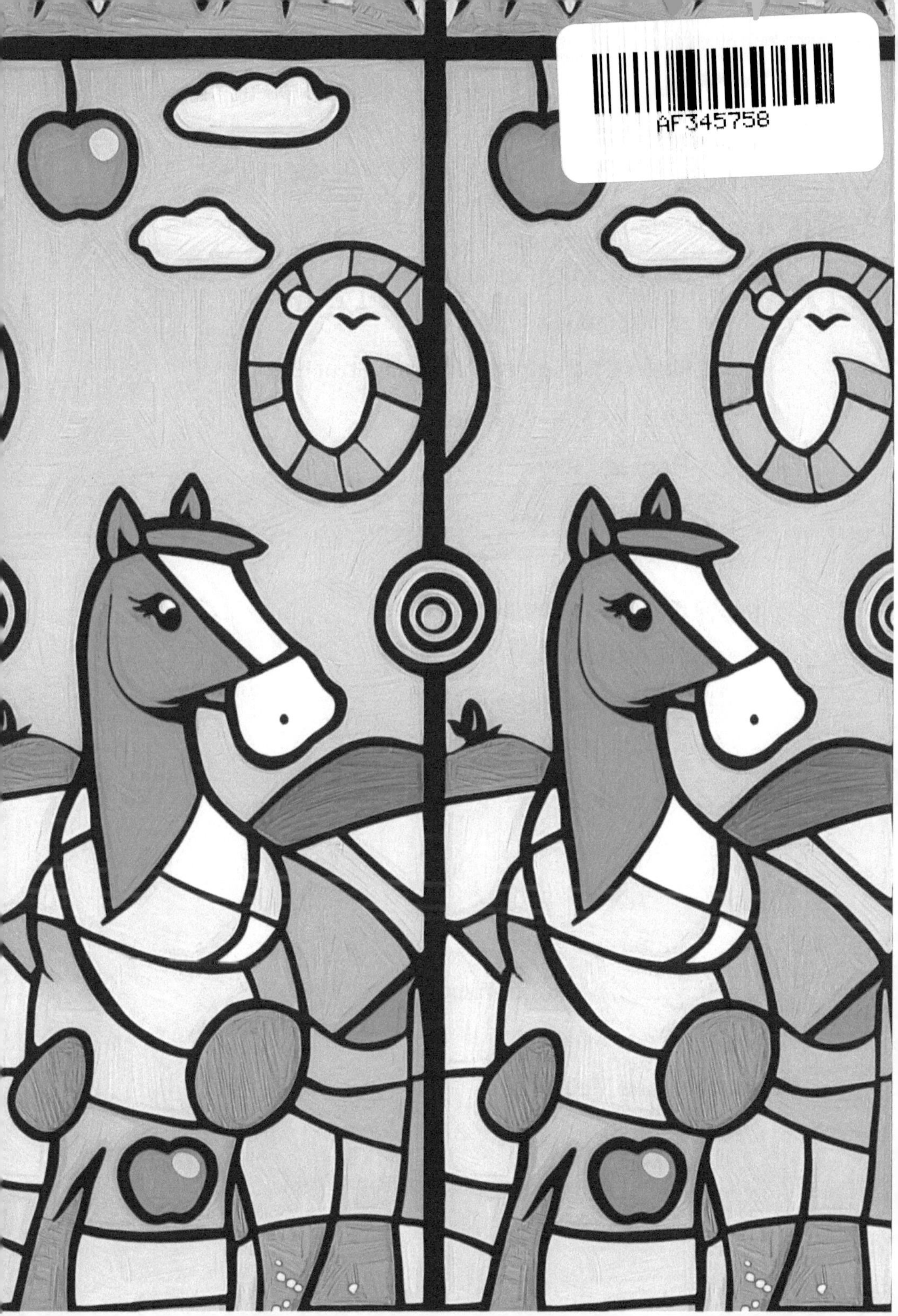
AF345758

Table of Contents

Artemis Saage

Horse Health:
A Complete Guide to Equine Anatomy and Natural Medicine

Master equine wellness through rehabilitation, massage, and science-based care - from basic anatomy to holistic healing methods

216 Sources
64 Photos / Graphics
23 Illustrations

Imprint

Saage Media GmbH
c/o SpinLab – The HHL Accelerator
Spinnereistraße 7
04179 Leipzig, Germany
E-Mail: contact@SaageMedia.com
Web: SaageMedia.com
Commercial Register: Local Court Leipzig, HRB 42755 (Handelsregister: Amtsgericht Leipzig, HRB 42755)
Managing Director: Rico Saage (Geschäftsführer)
VAT ID Number: DE369527893 (USt-IdNr.)

Publisher: Saage Media GmbH
Publication: 12.2024
Cover Design: Saage Media GmbH
ISBN Softcover: 978-3-384-43076-2
ISBN Ebook: 978-3-384-43077-9

Dear readers,

I sincerely thank you for choosing this book. With your choice, you have not only given me your trust but also a part of your valuable time. I truly appreciate that.

The health of your horse is the foundation for shared successes and harmonious coexistence. This practical handbook combines solid veterinary knowledge with proven natural healing methods. From detailed anatomy of the musculoskeletal system to specific instructions for first aid measures, you will gain a comprehensive insight into equine health. Benefit from the combination of conventional medical insights with alternative treatment methods such as herbal medicine and kinesiology taping. The book imparts practical knowledge for the prevention and treatment of common ailments— from muscle building to targeted support of the musculoskeletal system. With this guide, you will develop a deeper understanding of your horse's physical connections and be able to recognize health issues earlier. Strengthen your competence in horse care and build a valuable knowledge base for the optimal care of your four-legged partner.

I now wish you an inspiring and insightful reading experience. If you have any suggestions, criticism, or questions, I welcome your feedback. Only through active exchange with you, the readers, can future editions and works become even better. Stay curious!

Artemis Saage
Saage Media GmbH

- support@saagemedia.com
- Spinnereistraße 7 - c/o SpinLab – The HHL Accelerator, 04179 Leipzig, Germany

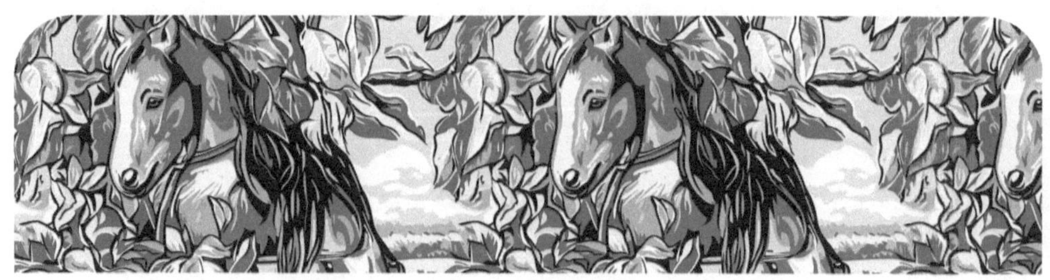

Introduction

To provide you with the best possible reading experience, we would like to familiarize you with the key features of this book. The chapters are arranged in a logical sequence, allowing you to read the book from beginning to end. At the same time, each chapter and subchapter has been designed as a standalone unit, so you can also selectively read specific sections that are of particular interest to you. Each chapter is based on careful research and includes comprehensive references throughout. All sources are directly linked, allowing you to delve deeper into the subject matter if interested. Images integrated into the text also include appropriate source citations and links. A complete overview of all sources and image credits can be found in the linked appendix. To effectively convey the most important information, each chapter concludes with a concise summary. Technical terms are underlined in the text and explained in a linked glossary placed directly below. For quick access to additional online content, you can scan the QR codes with your smartphone.

Additional bonus materials on our website
We provide the following exclusive materials on our website:

- Bonus content and additional chapters
- A compact overall summary
- A PDF file with all references
- Further reading recommendations

The website is currently under construction.

SaageBooks.com/horse_health-bonus-NSXJPU

1. Anatomy and Physiology of the Horse

How does the body of a horse function, and what makes it so special? This question occupies horse owners, veterinarians, and scientists alike. The horse's organism is a fascinating interplay of various systems—from the powerful musculoskeletal system to the highly specialized digestive tract and the finely tuned hormonal system. While evolution has shaped the horse into an enduring prey animal, we today impose entirely different demands on our four-legged partners. Whether as a sport horse, leisure companion, or therapy horse, understanding the anatomical and physiological foundations is essential for species-appropriate care, training, and medical treatment. How does the horse's body respond to different stresses? What role do hormones and metabolic processes play in health and performance? And how can we prevent diseases? The answers to these questions lie in a detailed examination of the various organ systems and their interactions. Only those who understand the fundamentals can recognize signs of illness early and respond appropriately. The following chapters provide a well-founded insight into the complex anatomy and physiology of the horse—from the basics to current scientific findings. This knowledge forms the foundation for all further aspects of equine health.

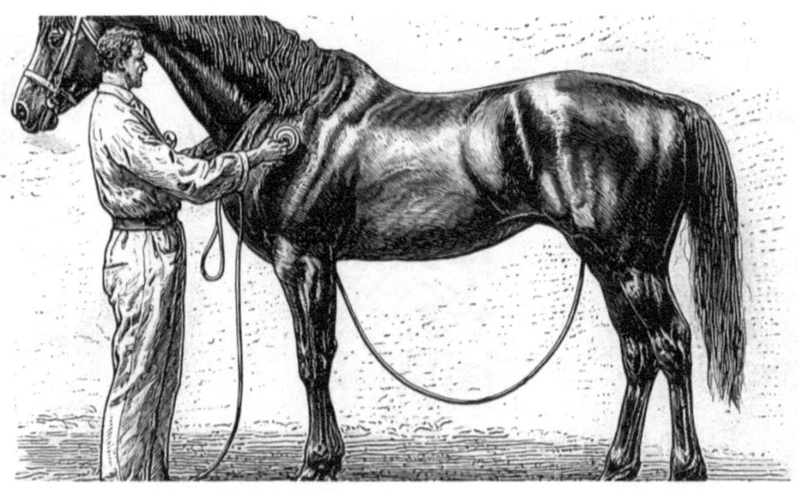

1. 1. Musculoskeletal System

he horse's locomotor system is a highly complex arrangement of bones, muscles, tendons, and ligaments that has perfectly adapted over millions of years to the demands of being a prey animal. How do these approximately 500 kg creatures manage to move both powerfully and gracefully? What mechanisms allow them to graze for hours and then, in the next moment, flee at lightning speed? The answers lie in the unique construction of the equine locomotor system: from the sophisticated hoof mechanism to the elastic spine, and the powerful muscles and tendons. Understanding these anatomical and physiological relationships is fundamental for anyone working with horses—be it as an owner, trainer, or therapist. Only those who comprehend the functioning of the locomotor system can recognize problems early and take appropriate preventive measures. The following chapters will illuminate the individual components of the locomotor system in detail and demonstrate how closely their interplay is linked to the horse's health.

„Musculoskeletal diseases are the most common diagnosis in equine medicine, with healing processes often not leading to complete regeneration, but rather resulting in inferior scar tissue."

1. 1. 1. Skeletal Structure and Bone Structure

he horse skeleton is a fascinating example of perfect adaptation for speed and strength. The bone structure is particularly rich in collagen, a protein that provides the bone with both stability and a certain degree of elasticity [s1]. This special composition allows horses to absorb enormous stresses during movement. Owners should therefore pay particular attention to a balanced calcium supply, especially during the developmental phase of young horses, as this forms the basis for healthy bone development. The collagen structure in horse bones changes significantly over the course of life. In young horses, there is a very dense and highly organized arrangement of collagen fibrils, which becomes looser and less structured with increasing age [s1]. This explains why older horses are often more susceptible to bone problems and should be trained more gently. A particularly important component of the musculoskeletal system is the articular cartilage (AC), which covers the ends of the joints [s2]. This special cartilage is structured in three zones, each fulfilling different functions. The superficial zone, with parallel collagen fibrils, ensures low-friction movements. Beneath it lies the middle zone with randomly oriented fibers, while in the deep zone, the fibrils run perpendicular to the joint surface. This sophisticated architecture, also known as Benninghoff architecture, develops during the maturation phase of the horse [s2]. The suspensory ligament, an evolutionary derivative of the middle intermuscular tendon, plays a central role in stabilizing the fetlock joint [s3]. It prevents excessive hyperextension and is therefore essential for maintaining the health of the limbs. Interestingly, the muscle composition in the suspensory ligament differs between the front and hind legs, with the front legs exhibiting a C-shaped and the hind legs a linear muscle arrangement [s3]. For trainers, it is important to know that Standardbreds have a higher muscle content in the suspensory ligament than Thoroughbreds, which should be taken into account when designing training programs. The biomechanical properties of articular cartilage are closely related to its composition [s2]. During movement, the cartilage distributes and mitigates the stresses that occur. To optimally fulfill this function, it contains not only collagen but also proteoglycans and chondrocytes. Riders should therefore pay particular attention to a progressive training design, especially for young horses, as the cartilage structure only fully develops during maturation. In practice, this means that particular care must be taken to gradually increase the load during the training of young horses, allowing the skeletal and cartilage tissues time to adapt. Regular, but moderate exercise is more important than intensive training sessions. For older horses, the declining stability of the collagen structure should be considered through adjusted training and, if necessary, supportive measures such as joint supplements. Maintaining the health of the musculoskeletal system also requires a balanced diet with sufficient minerals and trace elements. Especially during growth phases and in older horses, an adequate supply of bone-building substances is essential for maintaining skeletal health.

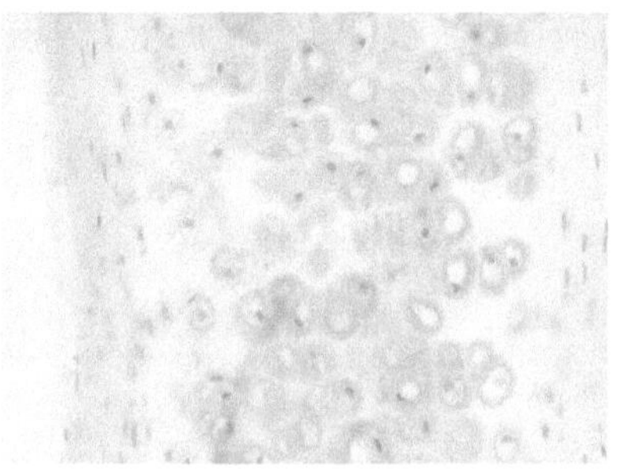

Chondrozyten [i1]

Glossary

Benninghoff Architecture
A three-dimensional structural principle of articular cartilage that
ensures optimal pressure distribution and stability through its
special fiber arrangement.

Chondrocyte
Specialized cells that live in small cavities within cartilage tissue
and are responsible for the production and maintenance of cartilage
substance.

Collagen
A fibrous protein that is the most important structural protein in the
body, making up about 30% of the total protein. It is primarily
responsible for the tensile strength of tissues.

Proteoglycan
Complex molecules made of proteins and sugar chains that can bind
water like a sponge, providing elasticity and compressive strength to
the tissue.

Suspensory Ligament
Also known as the fetlock supporter, it consists of elastic tissue and
is responsible for the cushioning of the horse's leg with each step.

1. 1. 2. Muscles and Tendons

he muscles and tendon tissue of the horse form a complex system that is crucial for movement, strength, and performance. Particularly, the <u>paraspinal</u> muscles along the spine play a central role in back health and can become overloaded due to injuries of the limbs or spine [s4]. This illustrates the close connection between various body regions in the horse's musculoskeletal system. Musculoskeletal diseases represent the most common diagnosis in equine medicine [s5]. A significant issue is that healing processes often do not lead to complete regeneration, resulting in inferior scar tissue. This explains the high rate of recurring injuries and underscores the importance of preventive measures. Horse owners should therefore pay particular attention to early signs of movement restrictions or behavioral changes that may indicate muscular problems. The development and maintenance of the <u>musculoskeletal</u> system is significantly influenced by the transcription factor <u>Sox9</u> [s6]. This factor regulates the development of muscles, tendons, and bones. A deficiency in Sox9 expression can lead to underdevelopment of these tissues. In practice, this means that particular attention must be paid to a balanced development of all structures, especially during the rearing and training of young horses. A systematic training approach with adequate recovery phases is essential. In the diagnosis and treatment of musculoskeletal disorders, chiropractic has established itself as an effective complementary method [s7]. It can help restore normal joint movement and relax tense muscles. Owners should ensure that the chiropractor has the appropriate qualifications and that treatment is always conducted in consultation with the attending veterinarian. Vertebral dysfunctions often manifest as local pain and muscle tension [s4]. A typical sign is the restricted mobility of certain body parts. Riders can often notice this through asymmetric movement or resistance during specific exercises. In such cases, a thorough examination by a specialist is indicated to avoid chronic damage.

The high rate of musculoskeletal injuries affects not only sport horses but also leisure horses [s5]. To prevent this, attention should be paid to balanced loading. This specifically means:
- Regular but moderate training
- Sufficient warm-up and cool-down phases
- Variation of training sessions
- Regular checks of equipment for proper fit
- Appropriate ground conditions during training

The still not fully understood mechanisms of tissue regeneration [s5] highlight the importance of prevention. A well-thought-out training management that considers the individual needs and training level of the horse is key to success. Regular check-ups by qualified professionals should also be scheduled to identify and address potential problems early.

Glossary

musculoskeletal
Refers to the interplay of muscles, bones, tendons, ligaments, and joints as a functional unit

paraspinal
Refers to the muscles running on both sides of the spine that are important for stabilizing and moving the spine

Sox9
A protein that acts as a genetic switch and particularly regulates the formation of cartilage and bone tissue during embryonic development

1. 1. 3. Hoof Mechanism

he hoof mechanism of the horse is a fascinating example of perfect adaptation to high loads. As a complex biomechanical system, the hoof consists of various structures that work together to absorb significant forces and utilize energy for forward movement [s8]. The outer hoof wall, which contains no blood vessels or nerves, bears the weight of the horse and protects the inner structures [s9]. It is covered with a special protective layer that prevents excessive moisture evaporation. In the absence of this layer, dryness and cracks can occur—a common problem in domesticated horses. Therefore, horse owners should regularly check the moisture balance of the hooves and use appropriate hoof care products as needed. A central element of the hoof mechanism is the expansion and contraction of the hoof during movement [s10]. With each step, the hoof expands laterally, facilitated by the digital cushion and the lateral cartilages. This flexibility is essential for shock absorption. In practice, this means that overly tight or rigid shoes can restrict this natural movement. Farriers should take this into account when selecting and applying shoes. The frog plays a special role in the hoof mechanism [s8]. It not only absorbs shocks but also supports the blood circulation of the hoof. The pressure on the frog compresses the blood vessels, acting like a natural pump and stimulating blood circulation in the leg [s11]. A healthy, well-developed frog is therefore crucial for overall hoof health. Horse owners should ensure that the frog is neither excessively trimmed nor damaged by consistently moist bedding during hoof care. Scientific studies have shown that the unshod hoof dampens vibrations better than the shod hoof [s12]. Shoeing reduces natural damping and increases the transmission of shocks to the first phalanx. This underscores the importance of carefully weighing whether and how a horse should be shod. Alternative methods such as hoof boots can be a sensible option in some cases.

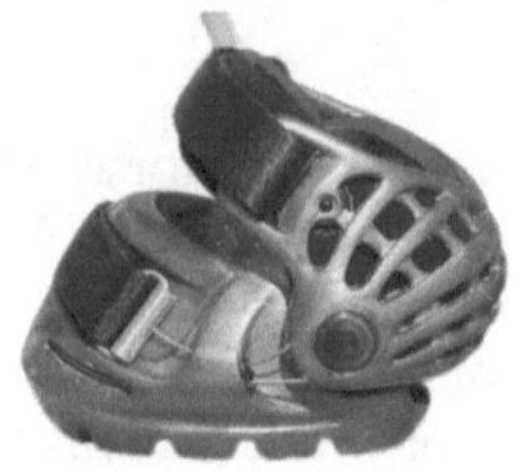

Hoof boots [i2]

Hoof growth typically amounts to about 0.6 to 1 cm per month [s13]. Interestingly, experiments with whole-body vibration plates have shown that they do not significantly accelerate hoof growth [s11]. In practice, this means that regular hoof care every 6-8 weeks is optimal for most horses. The sole of the hoof forms an important protective barrier between the ground and the inner structures [s14]. The coronary band, responsible for the growth of the hoof wall, is highly vascularized and should be protected from injuries. The inner hoof wall, with its lamellae, ensures a stable connection between the hoof wall and the coffin bone—a separation of this connection can lead to serious problems [s13].

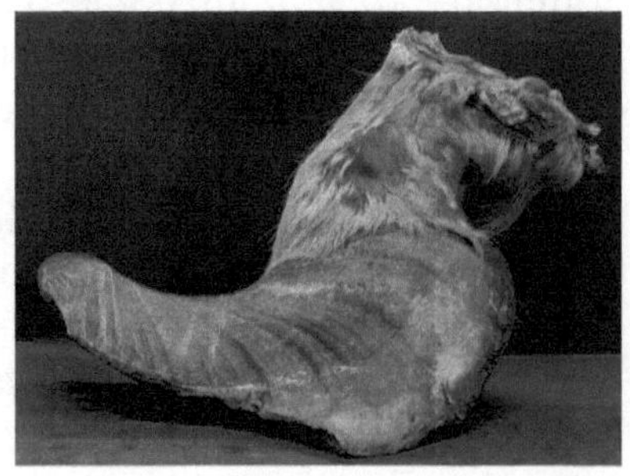

Hoof growth [i3]

For horse owners, it is essential to understand that the hoof mechanism can only function optimally if all components are healthy and can work naturally. In practice, this means:
- Regular professional hoof care
- Appropriate movement on various surfaces
- Clean, dry bedding
- Balanced nutrition for healthy horn growth
- Regular checks for signs of problems such as cracks or rot

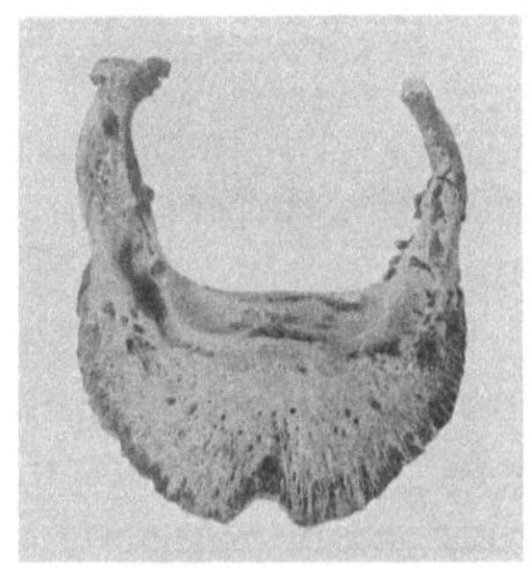

Hufpflege [i4]

Glossary

Lamella

Leaf-shaped tissue structures in the hoof that are arranged like interlocking fingers and provide stable suspension of the coffin bone within the horn capsule.

Phalanx

A limb bone in the horse that is part of the toe bones. The horse has three phalanges per leg, which, along with other bones, form the distal phalanx apparatus.

1. 1. 4. Spinal Function

he horse's spine is a masterpiece of evolution, fulfilling several vital functions simultaneously. With its five distinct sections - 7 cervical vertebrae, 18 thoracic vertebrae, 6 lumbar vertebrae, 5 sacral vertebrae, and a variable number of caudal vertebrae - it forms the central axis organ of the musculoskeletal system [s15]. Its significance extends far beyond mere support. One of the primary tasks of the spine is to protect the spinal cord, from which the nerve supply of the entire body is coordinated [s15]. The different shapes and orientations of the individual vertebrae allow for a complex interplay of various types of movement. It is important for riders to understand that mobility along the spine is not evenly distributed - the cervical region exhibits the greatest flexibility, while the lumbar region is significantly less mobile [s16]. The deep juxta-vertebral muscles play a crucial role in the stability of the spine. These highly innervated muscles surround several consecutive vertebrae and enable continuous adjustment of the spinal position [s16]. In practice, this means that well-developed back muscles are essential for maintaining the health of the spine. Riders should therefore pay particular attention to balanced conditioning of these muscle groups. Particularly interesting is the sophisticated ligament system of the spine. It allows the horse to lower its head without having to exert muscle power continuously [s16]. This explains why horses can graze relaxed with their heads lowered for extended periods. At the same time, this ligament system provides a biomechanical connection between the forehand and hindquarters. Scientific studies have shown that spinal movements between a straight and curved line differ significantly. When working in a circle, the lateral bending of the spine increases by about 3.6-3.75° [s17]. This insight is particularly relevant for training: riders should ensure that both sides are trained evenly to avoid unilateral strain.

The lumbar spine deserves special attention, as it must ensure both stability and flexibility. The five movable vertebrae allow movements in various planes, while the intervertebral discs between the vertebrae act as natural shock absorbers [s18]. For training practice, this means that exercises aimed at mobilizing and stabilizing this region are particularly important. The <u>dorsoventral</u> movements of the <u>thoracolumbar</u> intervertebral joints

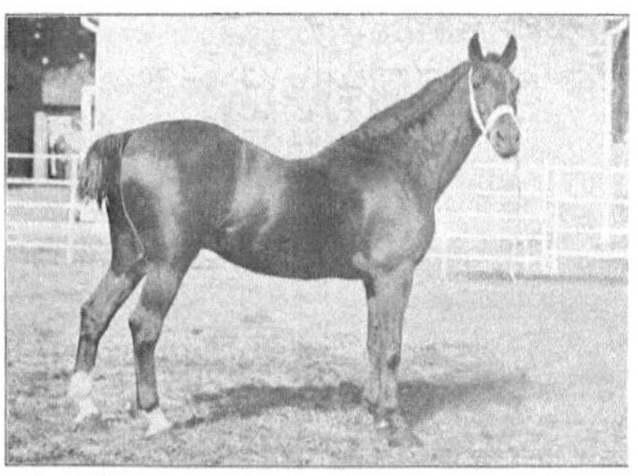

lumbar spine [i5]

follow a specific movement pattern that can be described as rotation around the center of the <u>caudal</u> vertebral body [s19]. This biomechanical insight aids in understanding back problems and their targeted prevention.

For horse owners and trainers, this results in important practical consequences:
- Regular monitoring of back muscles for tension
- Systematic development of carrying capacity through tailored training
- Balanced work on both reins
- Integration of stretching exercises into daily training
- Consideration of individual mobility restrictions
- Regular checks by qualified professionals

Maintaining the health of the spine requires a deep understanding of its function and appropriately adapted training design. Only when all involved structures - bones, muscles, ligaments, and nerves - work optimally together can the horse develop its full performance potential and remain healthy in the long term.

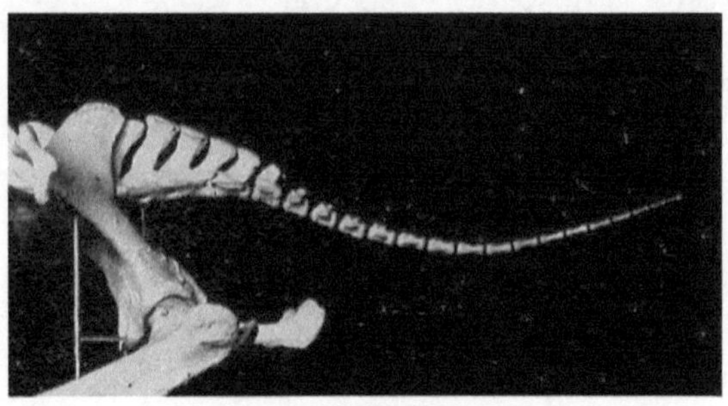

kaudalen Wirbelkörpers [i6]

Glossary

caudal
Anatomical directional term meaning 'located towards the tail'. In the context of the spine, it refers to the direction towards the horse's tail.

dorsoventral
Describes the direction from the back (dorsal) to the belly (ventral) or vice versa. This axis of movement is particularly important for the up and down movement of the horse's back.

juxta-vertebral
Refers to structures that lie directly next to the spine. This anatomical term originates from Latin, where 'juxta' means 'beside' or 'near'.

thoracolumbar
Refers to the transitional area between the thoracic and lumbar spine. This area is particularly relevant for the transfer of power between the forehand and hindquarters.

Summary - 1. 1. Musculoskeletal System

- The collagen in horse bones shows a highly organized arrangement of fibrils in young animals, which becomes looser with age.
- The articular cartilage is structured into three functional zones arranged according to the Benninghoff architecture.
- The suspensory ligament has a higher muscle component in Standardbreds than in Thoroughbreds.
- The paraspinal muscles can become overloaded due to limb or spinal injuries.
- The transcription factor Sox9 significantly regulates the development of muscles, tendons, and bones.
- The unshod hoof wall dampens vibrations better than the shod one.
- The frog acts as a natural pump for blood circulation in the leg.
- Whole-body vibration plates have no significant effect on hoof growth.
- The juxta-vertebral muscles allow for continuous adjustment of the spinal position.
- When working in a circle, the lateral bending of the spine increases by 3.6-3.75°.
- The dorsoventral movements of the thoracolumbar intervertebral joints rotate around the center of the caudal vertebral body.

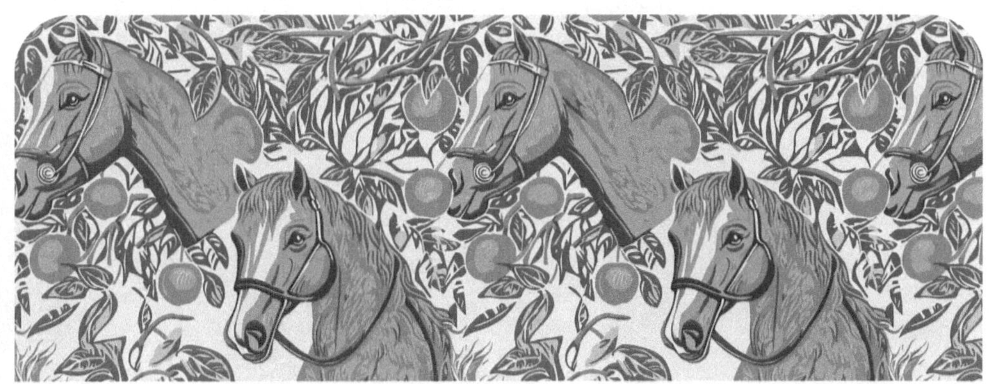

1. 2. Organ Systems

he complex organ systems of the horse form the foundation for its remarkable performance and health. But how do these various systems work together? What specific adaptations have developed over the course of evolution? And what significance do these peculiarities have for daily care and training? From the unique respiration as an obligate nasal breather to the highly specialized digestive tract and the powerful cardiovascular system—each organ system fulfills specific tasks and is in constant interaction with the other systems. The nervous system coordinates these complex processes, while the hormonal system fine-tunes the various bodily functions. Understanding these organ systems and their interconnections is not only relevant for veterinarians but also forms the basis for appropriate husbandry and effective health care. The following sections will illuminate the individual organ systems in detail and demonstrate how this knowledge can be applied in practice.

„*As obligate nasal breathers, horses can only breathe through their noses, as the pathway between the mouth and lungs is anatomically blocked.*“

1. 2. 1. Respiratory Organs

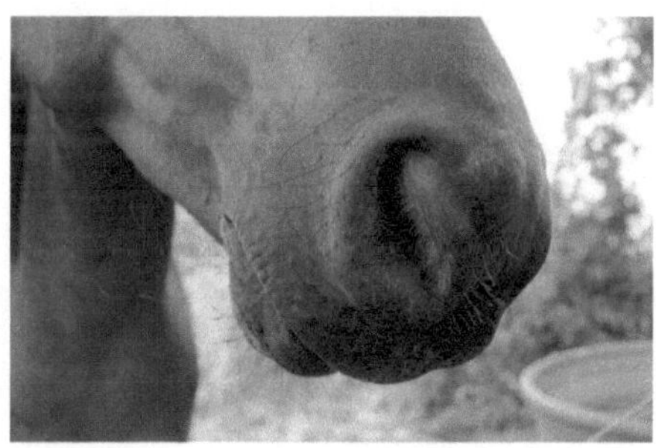he respiratory system of the horse is a highly complex and efficient organ system responsible for supplying the body with essential oxygen and expelling carbon dioxide [s20]. As obligate nasal breathers, horses can only breathe through their noses, as the pathway between the mouth and lungs is anatomically blocked—an important protective function that prevents food from entering the lungs [s21]. The respiratory tract is divided into an upper and a lower section [s22]. The upper respiratory tract begins with the nostrils, which, due to their movable cartilage structure, allow for optimal air intake, especially during intense exertion [s20]. Horse owners should therefore pay attention to the unrestricted mobility of the nostrils when examining their animals. The inhaled air then passes through the nasal cavities with their turbinates, the paranasal sinuses, the nasopharynx, and the larynx [s23]. In the nasal cavity, the inhaled air is warmed, moistened, and filtered by the richly vascularized mucous membrane [s24]. This preparation of the inhaled air is essential for maintaining the health of the sensitive lung structures. Stable owners should ensure a dust-free environment and good ventilation to avoid overwhelming the natural cleaning mechanisms. The lower respiratory tract consists of the trachea (trachea) and the lungs [s23]. The trachea is a flexible tube made of cartilage rings that branches into the bronchi [s20]. This structure can be prone to collapse during forced inhalation, which is why a veterinary examination is essential in case of respiratory issues.

Nostrils [i7]

The main function of the lungs is gas exchange in the <u>alveoli</u>, where oxygen is absorbed into the blood and carbon dioxide is expelled [s20]. This function is particularly crucial for athletic performance. Trainers should therefore always consider possible respiratory problems when their horses experience a decline in performance. Respiratory diseases can manifest through various symptoms: respiratory noises, decreased

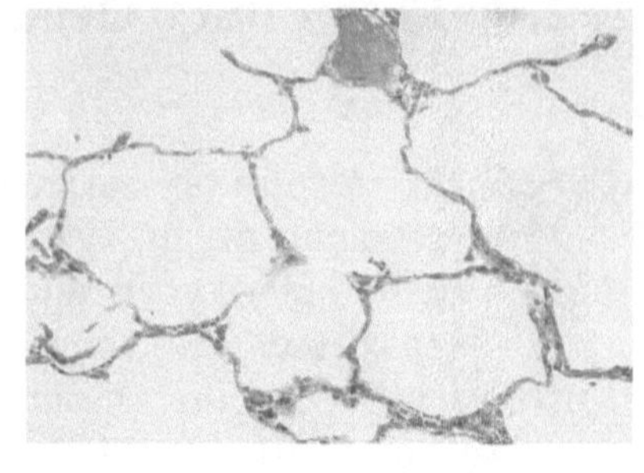

alveoli [i8]

performance, nasal discharge, bad breath, swelling in the face or neck, loss of appetite, elevated body temperature, and increased respiratory rate are important warning signals [s22]. In such cases, a veterinarian should be consulted immediately, who can employ various diagnostic procedures such as digital radiography, ultrasound, or endoscopy [s22]. The diseases can be of both infectious (viral or bacterial) and non-infectious nature [s23]. Preventive measures such as regular vaccinations, optimal stable hygiene, and adequate ventilation are therefore of great importance. Owners should also pay attention to dust-free bedding and high-quality, low-dust hay. The respiratory muscles, consisting of the diaphragm and intercostal muscles, are controlled by the autonomic nervous system [s20]. A healthy resting respiratory rate in adult horses is between 8-16 breaths per minute. Horse owners should regularly monitor this, as deviations can provide early indications of health problems.

Glossary

Alveolus

Microscopically small, grape-like air sacs with a total surface area of about 2500 square meters in adult horses.

Nasopharynx

An important connecting space between the nose and throat, approximately 15 cm long in horses, with a special mucous membrane lining.

Trachea

An approximately 70-80 cm long airway in adult horses, consisting of 50-60 horseshoe-shaped cartilage rings.

1. 2. 2. Digestive Tract

he digestive tract of the horse is a highly specialized system optimally adapted for the digestion of plant-based food. As herbivores and hindgut fermenters, horses possess anatomical and physiological features that enable efficient utilization of fiber-rich feed [s25]. Digestion begins in the mouth, where movable, strong lips and specialized teeth take in and break down the food [s25]. Horse owners should therefore ensure regular dental check-ups, as dental issues can significantly impair food intake. The chewed food is transported through the esophagus to the relatively small stomach, which holds only 8-16 liters [s26]. This limited capacity necessitates an adapted feeding strategy: instead of fewer large meals, several small portions should be offered throughout the day to prevent digestive disturbances [s27]. In the stomach, enzymatic digestion begins, supported by special structures such as <u>submucosal glands</u> along the greater curvature [s28]. The small intestine, consisting of <u>duodenum</u>, jejunum, and <u>ileum</u>, is the main site of nutrient absorption [s27]. The duodenum is fixed on the right side of the body by a short <u>mesentery</u>, which protects it from dislocation—an important anatomical adaptation [s26]. Particularly noteworthy is the significance of the hindgut for digestion. The cecum, with a capacity of about 30 liters, acts as a large fermentation tank [s26]. Here, microbial digestion occurs, where a complex community of bacteria and fungi breaks down plant fibers [s29]. These microorganisms produce essential B vitamins and volatile fatty acids, which cover 60-70% of the horse's daily energy requirements [s29]. To support this vital function, horse owners should ensure adequate roughage intake

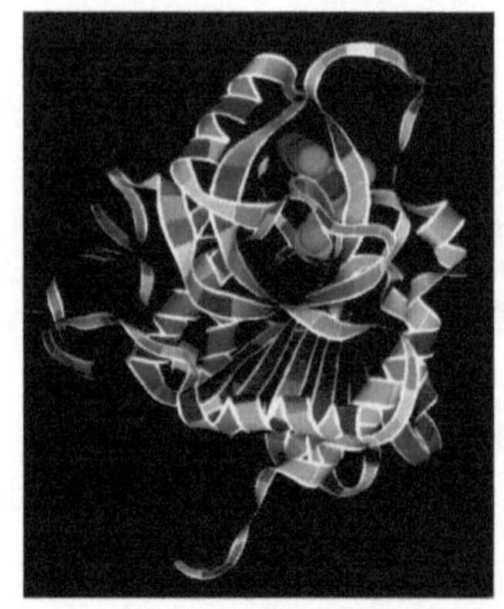

Enzyme [i9]

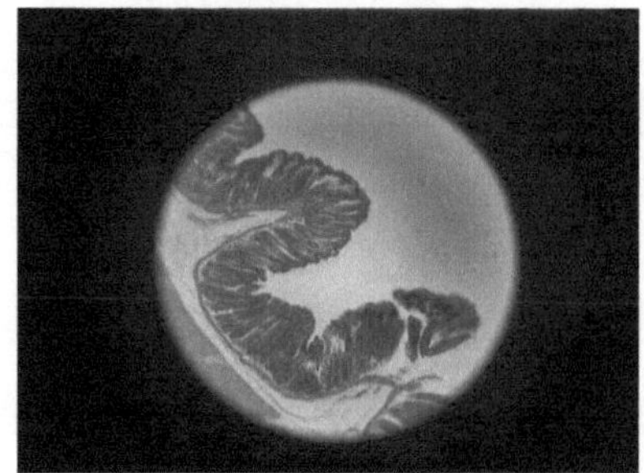

hindgut [i10]

and make dietary changes gradually. The large intestine, with its various sections—right and left ventral as well as dorsal colon—is a complex system where the food mass is fermented for 36-48 hours [s29]. The diversity of fungi is particularly pronounced in the hindgut, with anaerobic fungi playing a key role in breaking down cellulose [s30]. These microorganisms possess specialized enzymes (endoglucanases, exoglucanases, and β-glucosidases) that work synergistically to break down plant cell walls [s29]. Due to this complex anatomy, various digestive disorders can occur. The transition between the left ventral colon and the pelvic flexure is particularly susceptible to impactions [s26]. Therefore, horse owners should watch for signs such as reduced food intake, altered fecal output, or colic symptoms and seek veterinary assistance if in doubt. Nutrition has a significant impact on the composition of the gut microbiota and thus on digestive efficiency [s29]. A fiber-rich diet promotes the fibrolytic capacity of the intestine. Since the small horse stomach limits food intake, it may be necessary to supplement with concentrate feed during periods of high energy demand [s27]. However, this should always be done in small portions and with adequate chewing time in mind.

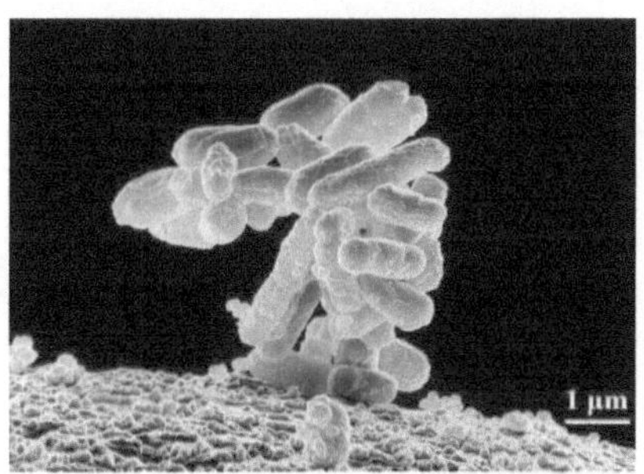

Microorganisms [i11]

Glossary

Duodenum
The first section of the small intestine, also known as the duodenum, which receives important digestive enzymes from the pancreas and bile from the liver.

Ileum
The last section of the small intestine, also known as the ileum, which is particularly important for the absorption of vitamin B12 and bile acids.

Jejunum
The middle section of the small intestine, also known as the jejunum, characterized by a particularly high number of intestinal villi for nutrient absorption.

Mesentery
A tissue structure made of connective tissue that suspends organs in the abdominal cavity and supplies them with blood vessels and nerves.

Submucosal Glands
Special glands located beneath the gastric mucosa that produce protective mucus and bicarbonate to shield the stomach wall from gastric acid.

1. 2. 3. Cardiovascular System

he horse's cardiovascular system is an impressive example of evolutionary adaptation to high athletic performance. With a heart that is approximately 13 times larger than that of an adult human [s31], the horse possesses an extraordinary cardiovascular capacity. This anatomical feature allows horses to quickly transition from resting phases to intense exertion situations. During training, the remarkable adaptability of the equine cardiovascular system becomes particularly evident. Oxygen uptake can increase by up to 35 times during submaximal exertion [s32]. The heart rate rises proportionally with the workload, without a decrease in stroke volume—an impressive feat considering that the heart rate can reach six to seven times the resting value during intense exertion [s32]. Various physiological mechanisms support this performance: spleen contraction releases additional red blood cells, venous return is enhanced, and the contractility of the heart muscle increases [s32]. An experienced trainer will optimally utilize these natural adaptive mechanisms through systematic conditioning training. The increase in workload should occur gradually to allow the cardiovascular system time to adapt. Interestingly, the equine cardiovascular system is relatively rarely affected by diseases compared to other organ systems [s33]. However, heart murmurs and arrhythmias can occur in riding horses [s34]. It is important for horse owners and trainers to know that not every heart murmur is pathological—the distinction between physiological and pathological sounds requires specialized veterinary expertise. Modern equine cardiology offers a wide range of diagnostic options. Veterinary cardiologists employ various examination methods, including <u>echocardiography</u>, <u>electrocardiography</u>, blood pressure measurement, and <u>Holter monitoring</u> [s35]. In cases of performance drops or noticeable behavioral changes, owners should not hesitate to seek a cardiological evaluation. Regular training leads to positive adaptations of the cardiovascular system. After a systematic training program, horses can achieve higher performance levels at the same submaximal heart rate [s32]. This is achieved, among other things, through improved <u>capillarization</u> of the muscles and more efficient oxygen diffusion. Trainers should therefore emphasize balanced conditioning training and use heart rate as an important parameter for workload management. Monitoring heart health should be part of routine health management. Early detection and appropriate treatment of heart diseases can significantly improve the horse's quality of life and life expectancy [s35]. Owners should integrate regular cardiological checks into their health care, especially for older horses or sport horses in intensive training. Particular attention should be paid to prevention. This includes a balanced diet, regular but not excessive exercise, and the avoidance of excessive stress. When working with the horse, sufficient warm-up and cool-down phases should be observed to gently adapt the cardiovascular system to the exertion and allow it to return to rest afterward.

Glossary

Capillarization
The formation of fine blood vessels in the tissue, enabling the exchange of oxygen and nutrients between blood and cells.

Echocardiography
An imaging ultrasound procedure for examining the heart, allowing real-time visualization of heart structures, valve function, and blood flow.

Electrocardiography
A method for recording the electrical activity of the heart, capable of detecting arrhythmias and heart muscle diseases.

Holter Monitoring
A portable long-term ECG recording over 24 hours or longer, capturing heart rhythm disturbances during the horse's normal daily activities.

1. 2. 4. Nervous System

The horse's nervous system is a highly complex control system that coordinates and regulates all bodily functions. As one of the primary organ systems, it, along with the musculoskeletal system and the digestive system, is particularly susceptible to diseases [s36].

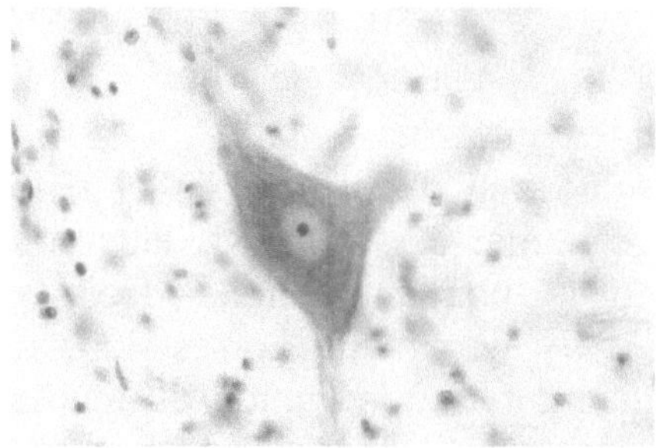

Nervous system [i12]

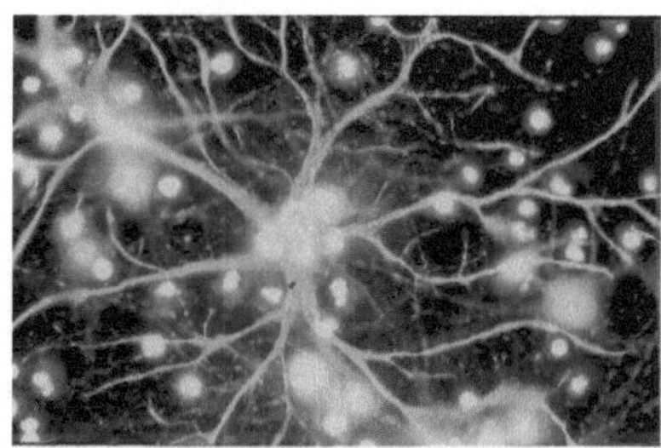

Astrocytes [i13]

A central role is played by the blood-brain barrier, which ensures controlled substance exchange between blood and brain. This barrier is formed by specialized <u>endothelial cells</u>, which prevent the uncontrolled passage of substances through particularly tight junctions [s37]. Horse owners should be aware that while this barrier is vital for life, it can also pose a challenge when administering medications, as not all active substances can cross this barrier. The nervous system is divided into the central

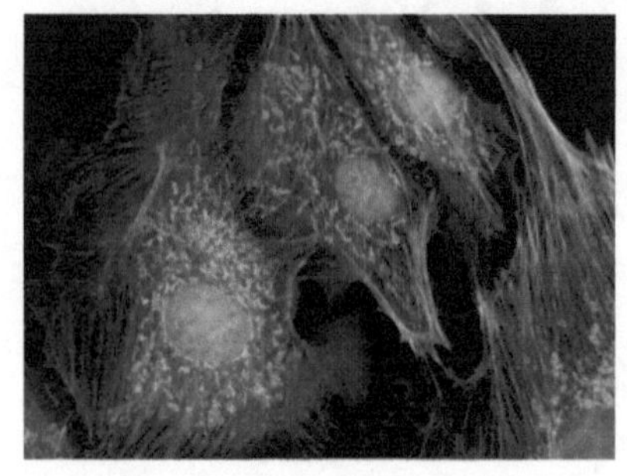

endothelial cells [i14]

nervous system (brain and spinal cord) and the peripheral nervous system with its twelve pairs of cranial nerves [s38]. This complex structure allows for the precise control of all bodily functions—from movement coordination to pain perception. In daily work with horses, it is important to watch for signs of neurological disorders: coordination difficulties, altered reactions to environmental stimuli, or unusual behavioral changes can be early warning signals. Particularly interesting is the role of the nervous system in pain processing. Targeted stimulation of nerves and nerve impulses can achieve pain relief [s39]. This is utilized, for example, in physiotherapy, where controlled forces are applied to elicit therapeutic responses through changes in joint structure and muscle function. The <u>astrocytes</u> and <u>pericytes</u> play an important role in maintaining the neurovascular unit [s37]. They assist the blood-brain barrier in regulating <u>ion homeostasis</u> and nutrient supply to the brain. It is crucial for horse owners to understand that disturbances in this delicate balance can lead to neurological symptoms. When assessing horse health, the neurological component should always be considered. Regular checks by a veterinarian can help detect neurological issues early. Special attention should be paid to the horse's coordination, balance, and responsiveness. The close relationship between spinal structure and neurological function [s39] underscores the importance of good back health for the entire nervous system. Therefore, horse owners should pay attention to proper saddle fitting and balanced training to avoid undue stress on the spine. Preventive measures such as regular exercise, a balanced diet, and avoidance of excessive stress can help maintain the health of the nervous system. In training and education, a gradual increase in demands should be observed to avoid overwhelming the nervous system.

Glossary

Astrocyte

Star-shaped cells in the brain and spinal cord that function as support cells and are involved in substance transport and signal transmission

Endothelial Cell

Specialized cells that line the innermost layer of blood vessels and selectively allow substances to pass through

Ion Homeostasis

Maintenance of a balanced ratio of electrically charged particles (ions) in the body

Pericyte

Small cells that surround blood vessels in the brain and regulate their permeability

1. 2. 5. Hormonal System

he hormonal system of the horse is a fascinating network of endocrine glands that communicate with each other through hormone signals in the blood, regulating vital bodily functions [s40]. The pituitary gland serves as the central control organ, regulating numerous metabolic and reproductive functions [s41]. The hypothalamic-pituitary-adrenal (HPA) axis and the thyroid axis (HPT) are of particular importance. These systems play a crucial role in stress responses and hormonal regulation [s42]. It is essential for horse owners to understand that chronic stress can disrupt these systems. Therefore, they should ensure a low-stress environment and a structured daily routine. As horses age, various endocrine disorders may arise. A common condition is pituitary dysfunction, which typically affects older horses [s40]. Symptoms are diverse and may manifest as changes in coat condition, chronic infections, increased sweating, as well as heightened thirst and urination. Attentive horse owners should consult a veterinarian upon noticing these signs. Another significant condition is equine metabolic syndrome, which bears similarities to metabolic syndrome in humans [s43]. It frequently occurs in middle-aged horses and is characterized by insulin resistance and increased body fat. The heightened risk of laminitis is particularly dangerous. Preventively, owners should focus on a balanced diet and regular exercise. The diagnosis of endocrine disorders is made through various hormone tests, noting that these are not always one hundred percent accurate [s40]. In cases of suspected pituitary dysfunction, the ACTH level is often measured [s41]. Treatment depends on the specific disorder—while pituitary dysfunction is usually treated pharmacologically with dopamine receptor agonists, the focus for metabolic syndrome is on adjusting diet and exercise [s43]. Interestingly, certain horse breeds show a genetic predisposition to endocrine disorders [s43]. Owners of these breeds should be particularly vigilant for early signs and take preventive measures if necessary. The hormonal system also plays a central role in regulating metabolism, growth, and digestion [s44]. For optimal function, a balanced diet is essential. Horse owners should ensure appropriate feeding and avoid obesity, as this increases the risk of hormonal disorders. An important aspect of hormonal regulation is urocortins (Ucns), which belong to the family of corticotropin-releasing hormones [s42]. They are detectable in various endocrine glands and influence various physiological processes through complex signaling pathways. These insights aid in understanding hormonal disorders and their treatment.

36

Glossary

ACTH
Adrenocorticotropic hormone - a hormone produced by the pituitary gland that stimulates the production of stress hormones in the adrenal glands.

Dopamine Receptor Agonist
Medications that mimic the action of the neurotransmitter dopamine and can thereby regulate certain hormone secretions.

Pituitary Gland
A hormone gland about the size of a hazelnut located at the base of the brain, also known as the master gland, which serves as the central control center for other hormone glands.

Urocortin
A group of signaling molecules that play a crucial role in stress adaptation and energy regulation, closely interacting with the immune system.

Summary - 1. 2. Organ Systems

- Horses are obligate nasal breathers, as the pathway between the mouth and lungs is anatomically blocked.
- The nasal cavity warms, moistens, and filters the inhaled air through highly vascularized mucous membranes.
- The trachea may tend to collapse during forced inhalation.
- The resting respiratory rate in adult horses is 8-16 breaths per minute.
- The small horse stomach holds only 8-16 liters, necessitating several small feed portions throughout the day.
- The cecum has a capacity of about 30 liters and functions as a fermentation tank.
- Volatile fatty acids from microbial digestion cover 60-70% of the daily energy requirement.
- The food bolus is fermented in the large intestine for 36-48 hours.
- The horse's heart is approximately 13 times larger than that of an adult human.
- Oxygen uptake can increase up to 35 times during submaximal exertion.
- Spleen contraction releases additional red blood cells during exertion.
- Astrocytes and pericytes support the blood-brain barrier in regulating ion homeostasis.
- The pituitary gland serves as the central control organ of the hormonal system.
- Urocortins influence various physiological processes through complex signaling pathways.
- Certain horse breeds exhibit genetic predispositions to endocrine disorders.

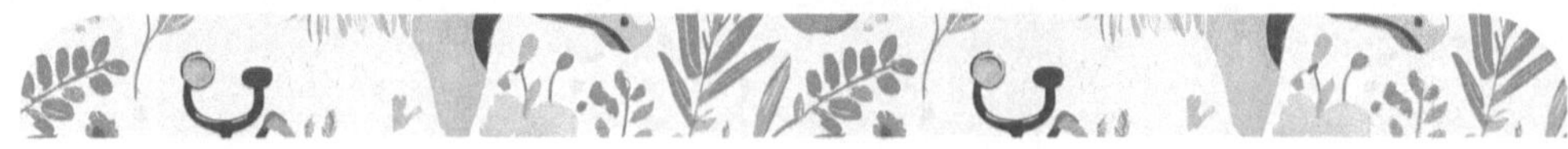

1. 3. Metabolic Processes

ow does the complex metabolism of a horse function, and what factors influence the various metabolic processes? What happens in a horse's body when it transitions between rest phases and sudden peak performance? These questions concern not only scientists but are also of great practical importance to horse owners. The metabolism of a horse encompasses a fascinating interplay of various systems—from energy balance to mineral metabolism, as well as vitamin supply and water regulation. Each of these areas follows its own principles yet is closely interconnected with the others. Disruptions in one area can have far-reaching consequences for the entire organism. Understanding these fundamental metabolic processes enables the proper nutrition of horses and helps prevent health issues. The following sections illuminate the individual aspects of metabolism and demonstrate how this knowledge can be applied in the daily practice of horse care.

„The metabolic flexibility of horses describes their ability to switch between different energy sources such as glucose and fatty acids—an important evolutionary adaptation that allows them, as prey animals, to quickly transition between rest and high-performance phases.“

1. 3. 1. Energy Balance

he energy balance of a horse is a complex system that significantly determines the health and performance of the animal. Metabolic flexibility plays a central role in this context—it describes the body's ability to switch between different energy sources such as glucose and fatty acids [s45]. This adaptability is particularly important, as horses, being prey animals, are evolutionarily designed to quickly alternate between rest and high-performance phases. A key enzyme in energy metabolism is the pyruvate dehydrogenase (PDC), which regulates the conversion of pyruvate into acetyl-CoA, thereby linking fat and sugar metabolism [s45]. In well-nourished, healthy horses, this enzyme operates with high activity. However, when less energy is consumed, its activity decreases to allow for glucose synthesis—a crucial adaptation mechanism for maintaining stable blood sugar levels. The microorganisms in the horse's stomach also play an important role in energy metabolism [s46]. They assist in breaking down nutrients and contribute to energy production. Interestingly, different horse breeds exhibit variations in their metabolic pathways, which should be considered in feeding practices. Exercise has a significant impact on energy balance. During physical activity, N-lactoyl-phenylalanine (Lac-Phe) is produced in greater amounts [s47], a signaling molecule that regulates food intake and counteracts obesity. This explains why regular exercise not only increases energy expenditure but also positively influences feeding behavior. For practical application, this means: 1. Feeding should be tailored to the individual situation of the horse. A competition horse has different energy needs than a leisure horse [s48]. As a rule of thumb: the higher the performance requirement, the more energy-dense the ration must be. 2. Regular exercise is essential for a healthy energy metabolism. Training sessions should be gradually increased to give the metabolism time to adapt [s49]. 3. When designing rations, metabolic flexibility must be taken into account. A balanced mix of carbohydrates and fats is important, with roughage forming the basis [s50]. Metabolic disorders such as insulin resistance can lead to metabolic inflexibility [s45]. In such cases, PDC activity is often impaired, leading to problems in energy utilization. Special feeding strategies are required to keep blood sugar levels as stable as possible. The neuroendocrine regulation plays an important role in controlling energy balance [s50]. Hormones such as insulin and glucagon coordinate energy storage and release. A disrupted hormonal balance can lead to metabolic issues.

For optimal energy management, it is recommended to:
- Regularly monitor body weight
- Adjust feed rations according to performance and health status
- Ensure sufficient exercise in all gaits
- Avoid long feeding breaks
- For performance horses: supplement with special energy feeds

Monitoring energy balance is particularly important for:
- Pregnant mares
- Growing foals
- Sport horses in intensive training
- Older horses
- Horses with metabolic diseases

A healthy energy balance is the foundation for the horse's performance and well-being. The interplay of feeding, exercise, and individual metabolic conditions must always be kept in mind.

Glossary

Metabolic Flexibility

An evolutionarily developed adaptability of metabolism that allows organisms to efficiently utilize different energy sources depending on availability.

Neuroendocrine Regulation

A complex interplay of the nervous and hormonal systems to control body functions. Occurs through specialized cells that function as both nerve cells and hormone-producing cells.

N-lactoyl-phenylalanine

A signaling molecule produced during physical activity from the amino acid phenylalanine and lactic acid. Plays an important role in appetite regulation after exercise.

Pyruvate Dehydrogenase

An enzyme complex consisting of several subunits located in the mitochondria of cells. Disturbances in this enzyme can lead to severe metabolic diseases.

1. 3. 2. Mineral Metabolism

he mineral metabolism in horses is a complex system responsible for numerous vital functions in the body. Although minerals constitute only a small part of the diet, they are involved in nearly all physiological processes and are indispensable components of amino acids, hormones, and vitamins [s51].

The interplay between calcium and phosphorus is particularly important. Calcium, of which 99% is found in the skeleton [s52], must be ingested in a ratio of approximately 1.5:1 to phosphorus [s53]. A practical example illustrates the significance: A 500 kg horse requires about 30g of calcium and 20g of phosphorus daily. While the calcium requirement can usually be met through high-quality hay, targeted mineral supplementation is often necessary during intense use or growth. The <u>electrolytes</u> sodium and potassium play a central role in regulating fluid balance and nerve impulse transmission [s54]. During heavy sweating, for example after intense training or on hot summer days, horse owners should pay particular attention to electrolyte supply. A practical tip: After strenuous work, an electrolyte paste or solution can be administered to compensate for losses.

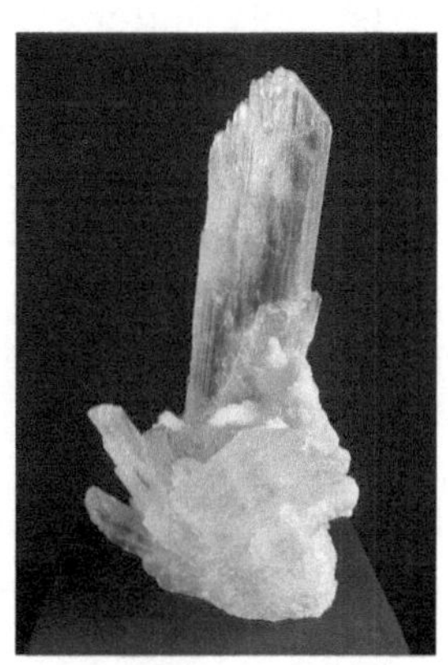

Calcium [i15]

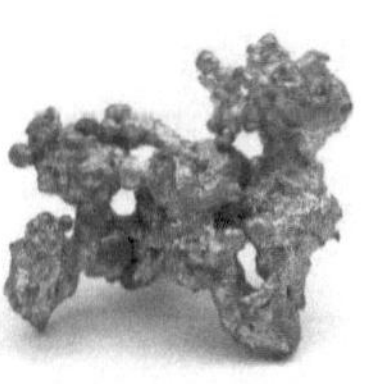

Copper [i16]

Trace elements such as zinc, copper, manganese, and selenium are essential for various metabolic processes [s55]. Zinc, for instance, supports hoof and coat quality, while copper is important for the immune system [s53]. A deficiency often manifests only after weeks or months, such as through brittle hooves or dull coats. Therefore, regular monitoring of mineral supply is advisable, especially for:
- Breeding horses
- Sport horses in training
- Horses with metabolic disorders
- Senior horses

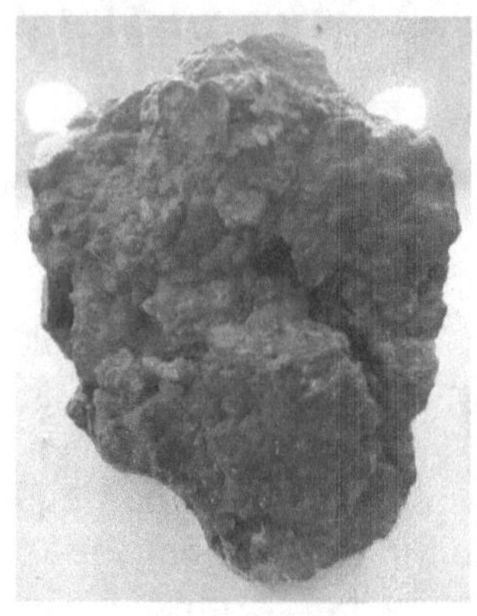

Manganese [i17]

The bioavailability of minerals plays a crucial role. Interestingly, alfalfa has been shown to possess particularly good biosorption properties for various minerals [s51]. This makes it a valuable component in horse feeding, especially for horses with increased mineral needs. Iodine is another important trace element required for the production of thyroid hormones T3 and T4 [s53]. These hormones regulate the metabolic rate of the entire organism. A practical note: In iodine-deficient areas, attention should be paid to adequate supplementation.

For optimal mineral supply, the following is recommended:
- Regular analysis of the base feed used
- Adjustment of mineral supplementation to individual needs
- Consideration of regional conditions (e.g., selenium-deficient soils)
- Attention to interactions between different minerals

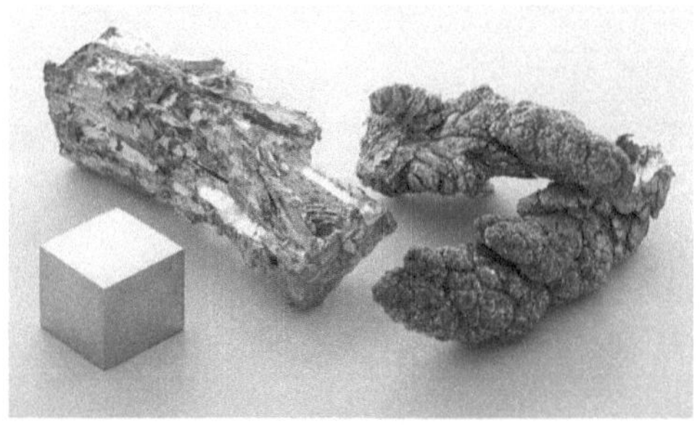

Zinc [i18]

Vitamin D plays a special role in mineral metabolism, as it regulates the absorption of calcium and phosphorus from the intestine and their incorporation into the skeleton [s52]. Sufficient sunlight is important for the activation of the vitamin. A practical piece of advice: Horses should have daily access to outdoor areas, ideally even on overcast days. Cobalt is another essential trace element needed for the formation of vitamin B12 by the gut flora [s53]. This underscores the importance of a healthy gut flora for overall mineral metabolism.

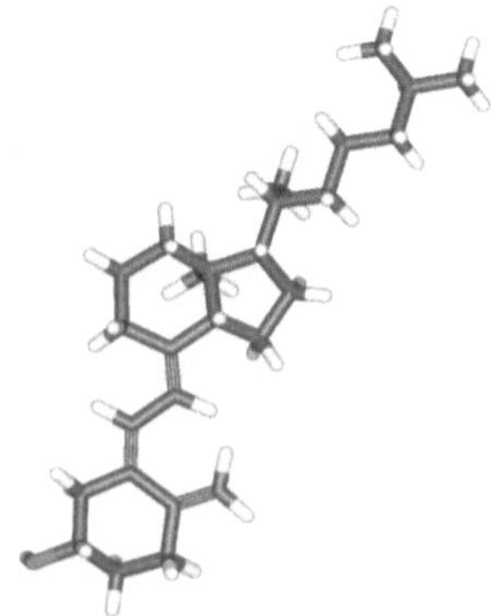

Vitamin D [i19]

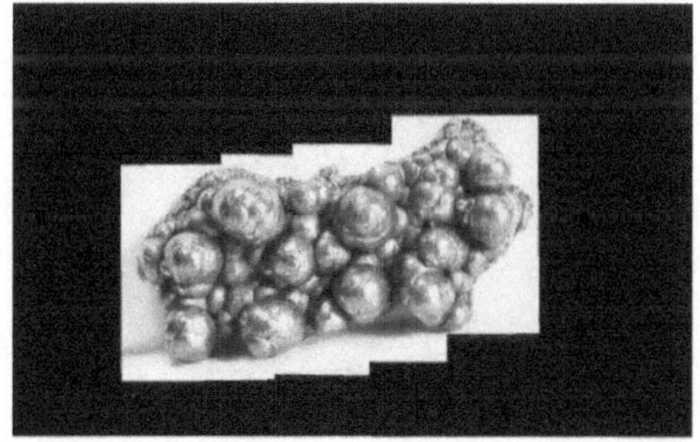

Kobalt [i20]

Glossary

Biosorption
A natural process in which certain materials or organisms can absorb and bind substances from their environment. In plants, it refers to the ability to efficiently take up nutrients from the soil.

Electrolyte
Mineral compounds that dissociate into electrically charged particles in water. They are essential for muscle contraction and water distribution in the horse's body.

1. 3. 3. Vitamin Requirements

he vitamin requirements of horses are closely linked to their health and performance. Particularly, vitamin E plays a central role as an essential nutrient for neuromuscular function [s56]. As a primary antioxidant, it prevents lipid peroxidation and stabilizes plasma membranes [s57]. The recommended daily dose is 1-2 international units per kilogram of body weight, with maintenance requirements at 50 IU/kg dry matter intake and growth requirements at 80 IU/kg [s57]. Fresh green forage is the best natural source of vitamin E; however, its content drastically decreases during the drying process to hay [s56]. Therefore, horse owners should pay particular attention to adequate supplementation, especially in stable housing. A practical tip: Before starting supplementation, a blood test is advisable, as some horses may have an increased requirement due to genetic variations [s56].

The absorption of vitamin E occurs passively through intestinal cells and depends on sufficient fat intake [s57]. The liver plays a key role in this process—the α-tocopherol transfer protein selectively binds RRR-α-tocopherol and packages it into lipoproteins for transport in the body [s57]. Vitamin K is essential for blood coagulation, vascular health, and bone metabolism [s58]. Interestingly, a primary vitamin K deficiency has never been observed in horses, as intake through feed and production by gut bacteria is usually sufficient. However, supplementation may be beneficial in cases of pure stable housing without access to fresh green forage [s58]. The requirement for vitamin A is closely linked to metabolism, vision, fertility, and the immune system [s59]. It supports the body's adaptability to physical stress—particularly important for sport horses. A practical note for competition riders: After intense training, special attention should be paid to vitamin E supply, as it supports recovery [s59]. B vitamins play a central role in energy metabolism and nerve function [s59]. Thiamine, riboflavin, niacin, pantothenic acid, pyridoxine, biotin, folic acid, and cyanocobalamin form a complex network. Vitamin C, as an important antioxidant, supports the immune system and is involved in the formation of healthy connective tissues [s59]. Particular attention should be paid to vitamin E supply in the first year of life, as a deficiency has been associated with the development of neuroaxonal dystrophy and degenerative myeloencephalopathy [s60]. Affected animals have shown an increased metabolic rate of α-tocopherol, highlighting the necessity for high-dose supplementation in genetically susceptible animals [s60].

The following recommendations arise for practice:
- Regular turnout for natural vitamin supply
- Supplementation in stable housing or increased need
- Blood value monitoring before starting supplementation
- Special attention to vitamin supply in:

* Young horses in growth
* Sport horses in intensive training
* Breeding mares
* Horses without access to pasture

A deficiency in vitamin E can manifest through various neuromuscular diseases [s56]. Risk factors include lack of pasture access, inadequate dietary supply, or excessive copper in the diet [s61].

α-tocopherol [i21]

Glossary

Lipid Peroxidation

A damaging chemical process in which free radicals can attack and destroy fatty acids in cell membranes.

Myeloencephalopathy

A disease that affects both the spinal cord and the brain, potentially leading to neurological deficits.

Neuroaxonal Dystrophy

An inherited disease of the nervous system in horses that leads to movement disorders and coordination problems.

α-Tocopherol

The biologically most active form of vitamin E, which can be particularly well absorbed and utilized by the body.

1. 3. 4. Water Balance

he water balance in horses is a finely regulated system responsible for numerous vital functions in the body. An adult horse weighing 500 kg consists of approximately 65% water, which corresponds to a total water volume of around 325 liters [s62]. This impressive amount underscores the central importance of water balance for the horse's health. Under normal conditions, a 500 kg horse requires about 27-30 liters of water daily, with approximately 85% being consumed through direct drinking [s62]. The remainder is provided through food and metabolic water. A practical tip for horse owners: daily water intake should be monitored, as sudden changes in drinking behavior may indicate health issues. Particularly during physical exertion or at high temperatures, the water requirement significantly increases. Horses can lose astonishing amounts of fluid during training—5-7 liters per hour under moderate conditions, and even up to 10-12 liters during extreme exertion [s62]. This highlights why water supply is especially important during athletic activity. A fascinating aspect of equine physiology is the ability to partially compensate for water loss through fluid reserves from the gastrointestinal tract [s62]. This evolutionary adaptation allows horses to endure longer periods of exertion. Nevertheless, horse owners should remain vigilant: clinically relevant dehydration occurs when a horse loses 3% or more of its body mass due to fluid loss [s63]. Sweat production in horses is significantly higher compared to humans, leading to substantial electrolyte loss [s63]. A practical note for competition riders: after intense training, not only water but also a balanced electrolyte supplement should be provided. Solely giving water without electrolytes can even exacerbate dehydration [s64].

The following important recommendations arise for practice:
- Constant access to fresh, clean water
- Regular checks of water troughs for functionality
- Additional water offerings in heat or during intense work
- Electrolyte supplementation after heavy sweating
- Monitoring drinking behavior as a health indicator

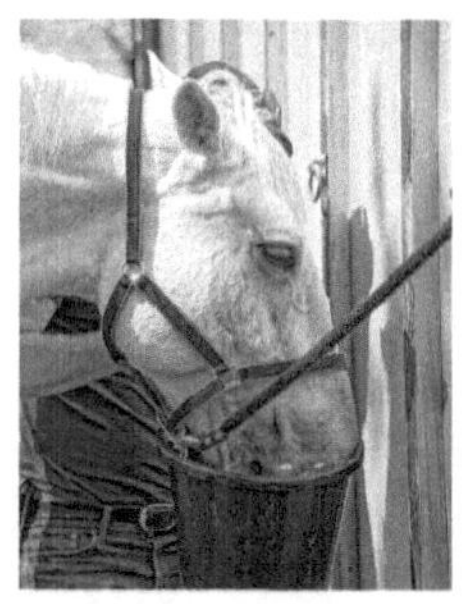

Water balance [i22]

Water balance is closely linked to acid-base equilibrium and kidney function [s65]. Intense exercise affects the blood viscosity and can lead to changes in plasma aldosterone concentration, which in turn influences renal sodium excretion [s65].

Particular attention should be paid to water balance in:
- Sport horses in intensive training
- Horses in high ambient temperatures
- Pregnant mares
- Older horses
- Horses with health limitations

An important practical aspect is monitoring hydration. The following signs may indicate dehydration:
- Delayed skin fold return
- Dry or sticky mucous membranes
- Sunken eyes
- Decreased urine output
- Dark-colored urine

Water supply should be ensured, especially during transport and competitions. A practical tip: many horses prefer to drink from familiar containers or prefer water from home. It may therefore be sensible to bring one's own water when traveling or to mix a little apple juice with unfamiliar water to increase acceptance.

Glossary

Blood Viscosity
Describes the thickness of the blood, determined by the proportion of solid components such as red blood cells. Increased viscosity can hinder circulation.

Plasma Aldosterone
A hormone of the adrenal cortex that regulates mineral balance and is particularly important for maintaining sodium-potassium equilibrium in the body.

Summary - 1.3. Metabolic Processes

- Pyruvate dehydrogenase regulates the conversion of pyruvate to acetyl-CoA, thereby linking fat and carbohydrate metabolism.
- During physical activity, N-lactoyl-phenylalanine is produced, which regulates food intake.
- Different horse breeds exhibit variations in their metabolic pathways.
- 99% of the calcium in a horse's body is found in the skeleton.
- Alfalfa demonstrates particularly good biosorption properties for various minerals.
- The vitamin E content in green forage drastically decreases during the drying process to hay.
- The absorption of vitamin E occurs passively through intestinal cells and requires adequate fat intake.
- The α-tocopherol transfer protein in the liver selectively binds RRR-α-tocopherol for transport.
- A primary vitamin K deficiency has never been observed in horses.
- Vitamin E deficiency is associated with the development of neuroaxonal dystrophy and degenerative myeloencephalopathy.
- A 500 kg horse is composed of approximately 65% water (325 liters).
- Horses can lose 5-7 liters of fluid per hour during training, and up to 10-12 liters under extreme exertion.
- Clinically relevant dehydration occurs with a 3% loss of body mass due to fluid loss.
- Intense exercise affects blood viscosity and plasma aldosterone concentration.

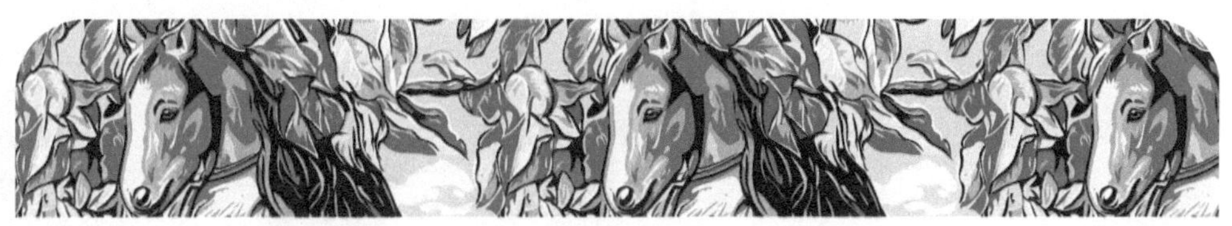

Review - 1. Anatomy and Physiology of the Horse

- The horse skeleton contains particularly high levels of collagen for stability and elasticity. The collagen structure in the bone becomes looser and less structured with increasing age. The articular cartilage is composed of three zones with collagen fibrils arranged differently. The suspensory ligament stabilizes the fetlock joint and prevents excessive hyperextension. Standardbreds have a higher muscle content in the suspensory ligament than Thoroughbreds. Musculoskeletal diseases are the most common diagnosis in equine medicine. The transcription factor Sox9 regulates the development of muscles, tendons, and bones. The unshod hoof dampens vibrations better than the shod hoof. The blood-brain barrier is formed by specialized endothelial cells with particularly tight junctions. Astrocytes and pericytes assist the blood-brain barrier in regulating ion homeostasis. The pituitary gland regulates numerous metabolic and reproductive functions. During exercise, oxygen uptake can increase by up to 35 times. Heart rate rises proportionally with workload, without a decrease in stroke volume. A 500 kg horse is composed of approximately 65% water (325 liters). Horses can lose 5-7 liters of fluid per hour during exercise. Metabolic flexibility allows for rapid switching between different energy sources. Lac-Phe is produced during physical activity and regulates food intake. Calcium and phosphorus must be ingested in a ratio of about 1.5:1. Alfalfa exhibits particularly good biosorption properties for various minerals. Vitamin E is essential for neuromuscular function and prevents lipid peroxidation.

- While these anatomical and physiological foundations form the basis for understanding equine health, natural healing methods offer fascinating possibilities to gently support and balance these complex systems.

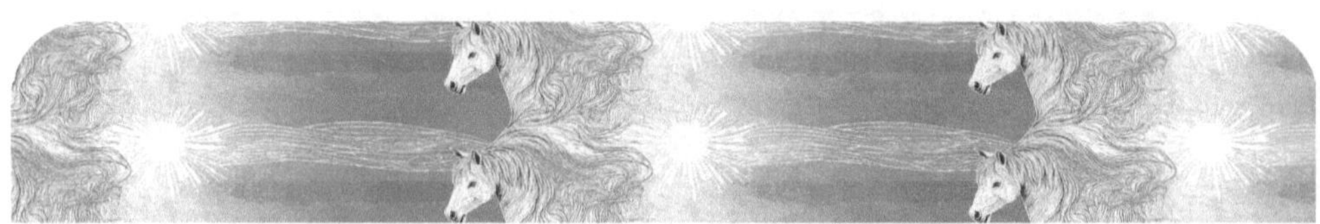

2. Natural Healing Methods

Natural healing methods have fascinated humanity for millennia. But what role do they play today in modern equine medicine? Can traditional healing practices such as acupuncture, osteopathy, or phytotherapy meaningfully complement conventional veterinary medicine? The growing importance of holistic therapeutic approaches raises important questions: How can the effectiveness of natural healing methods be scientifically demonstrated? Which methods are particularly suitable for the treatment of horses? And what are the limitations of natural medicine? This chapter explores various natural healing methods and their application in equine medicine. Both traditional practices and modern developments are presented and critically evaluated. A particular focus is placed on practical implementation and integration into existing treatment concepts. The increasing scientific exploration of natural healing methods opens new perspectives for evidence-based complementary equine medicine. The combination of established natural healing practices with modern veterinary medicine could pave the way for a more holistic health care approach for our horses.

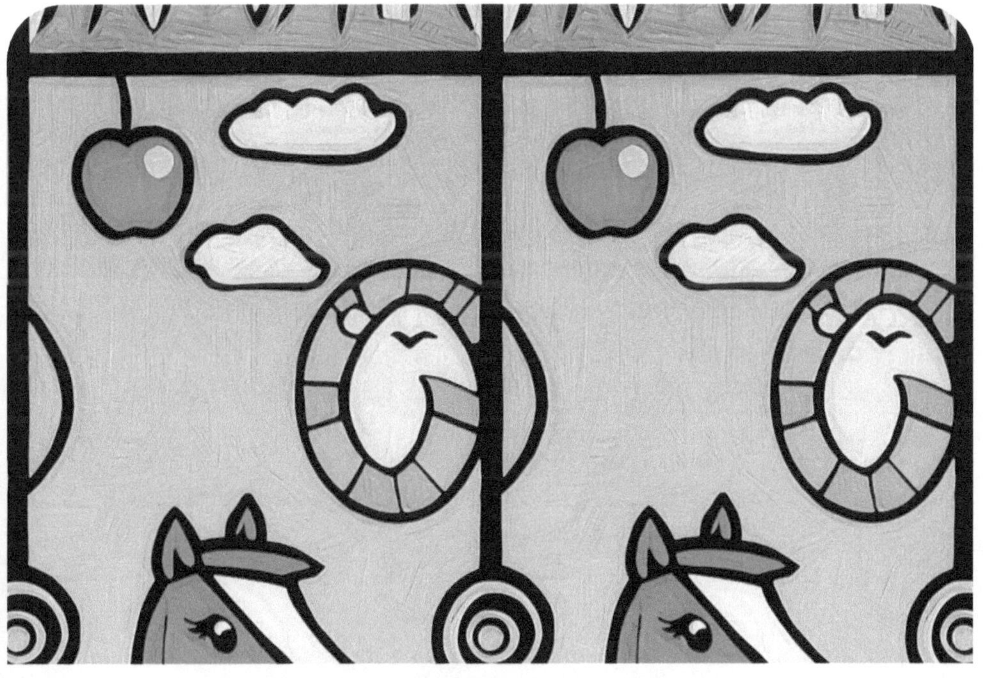

2. 1. Herbal Medicine

he use of medicinal herbs in equine medicine raises intriguing questions: How can traditional healing plants meaningfully complement modern veterinary medicine? What scientific findings confirm the efficacy of herbal remedies for various equine ailments? Herbology combines centuries-old experiential knowledge with current research results. It becomes evident that many medicinal plants contain bioactive substances that demonstrably exert therapeutic effects—whether in respiratory diseases, digestive issues, or in supporting the immune system. Specific plant compounds can also positively influence healing in wound treatment. The targeted application of medicinal herbs requires a solid understanding of their effects, dosages, and potential interactions. Recent scientific studies provide new insights into the complex mechanisms of action of plant ingredients and their therapeutic potential in equine medicine.

„Thyme contains essential oils with mucolytic and antibacterial properties and is used in horses at about 2-3 g of dried herb per 100 kg of body weight as a feed additive or hay infusion.“

2. 1. 1. Healing Herbs for Respiratory Tract

n horses, respiratory diseases play a significant role, as these animals, being former steppe dwellers, are particularly sensitive to stable conditions and the associated environmental influences [s66]. The targeted use of healing herbs can provide support and significantly improve the well-being of the animals.

Various traditional healing herbs have proven particularly effective, having been used in equine medicine for centuries. Thyme, for example, contains essential oils with mucolytic and antibacterial properties. In practice, it has been effective to add thyme to the feed or to spray it as an infusion over hay. Approximately 2-3 grams of dried herb should be used per 100 kg of body weight.

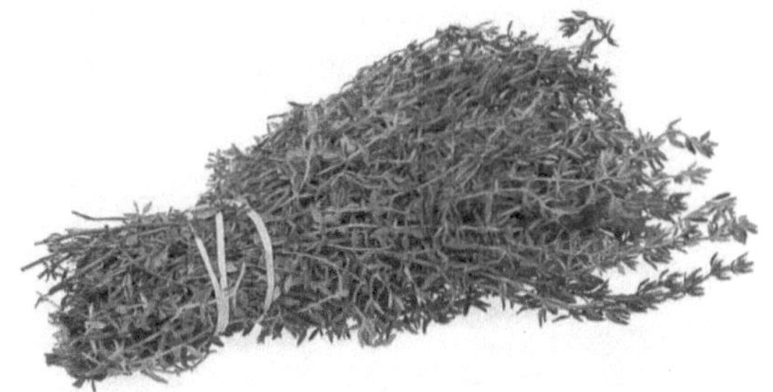

Thyme [i23]

Eucalyptus is another important healing herb for the respiratory tract. Its strong disinfectant and mucolytic properties make it a valuable aid for blocked airways. In application, inhalation is particularly recommended: hot water with a few drops of eucalyptus oil is prepared in a bucket and offered to the horse for inhalation for about 10-15 minutes [s66]. A promising new approach in the treatment of respiratory diseases is the use of water-soluble curcumin. Scientific studies have shown that this substance can reduce the production of harmful oxygen compounds

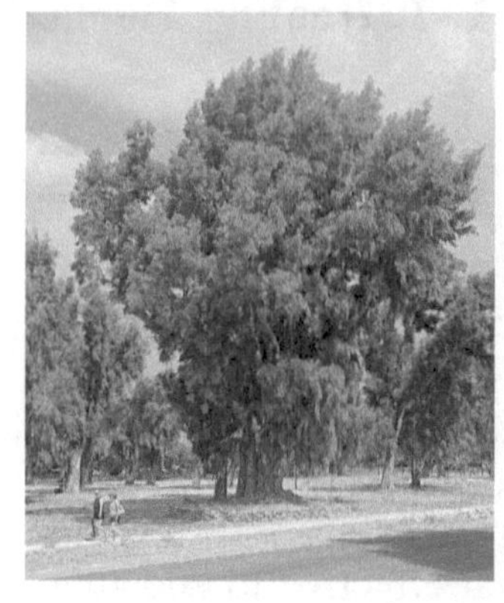

Eucalyptus [i25]

due to its anti-inflammatory properties [s67]. The administration through inhalation is particularly effective, with the water-soluble form exhibiting significantly better bioavailability than conventional curcumin.

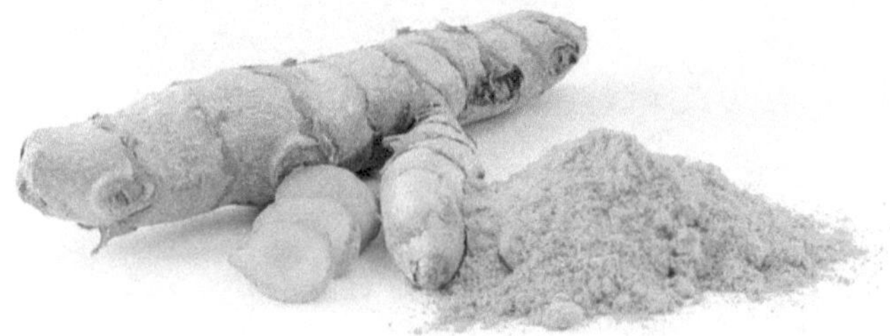

Curcumin [i24]

Mint and fennel are other well-established healing herbs that can be effectively combined. While mint clears the airways with its cooling effect, fennel supports mucus dissolution. In practical application, both herbs can be brewed as tea and used for inhalation or mixed into drinking water.

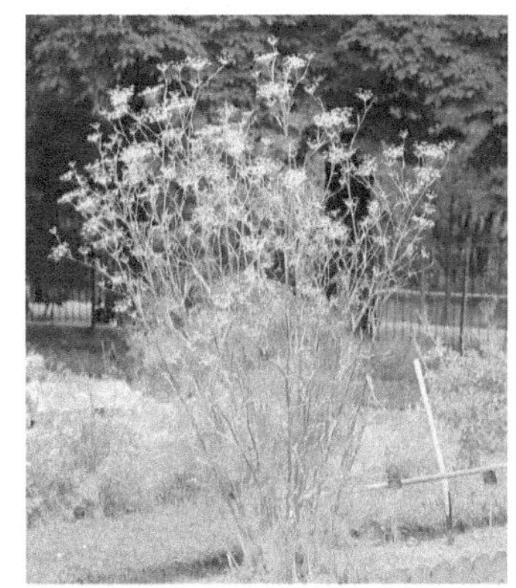

Fennel [i26]

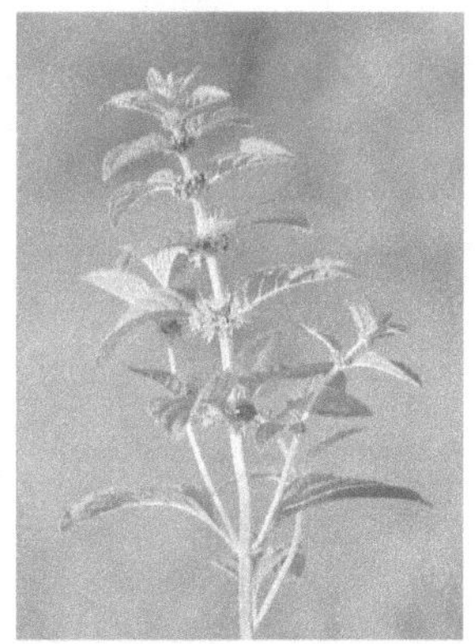

Mint [i27]

Sage has proven particularly effective in treating acute irritative conditions of the respiratory tract. Its antibacterial effect makes it a valuable aid in the early stages of infections. In practice, administering it as a tea infusion mixed with feed has been effective.

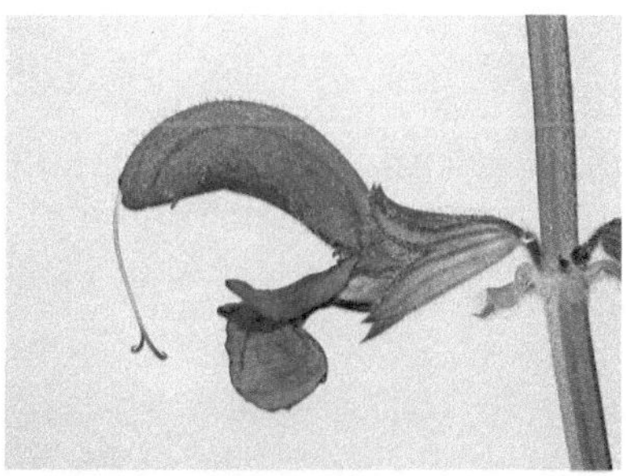

Sage [i28]

Anise rounds out the spectrum of respiratory herbs and is especially valued for its antispasmodic properties. It can be well combined with other herbs and enhances their effects [s66]. When using healing herbs, it is important to observe some basic rules. The dosage should always be adjusted to the horse's weight. Additionally, herbs should not be used continuously but rather in courses of 2-3 weeks. Especially in cases of chronic diseases, it is advisable to discuss treatment with a veterinarian [s66]. Research findings on the effects of water-soluble curcumin show promising results: treatment led to a significant reduction in inflammatory markers in bronchial fluid without affecting the number of defense cells [s67]. This suggests that curcumin specifically intervenes in inflammatory processes while not impairing the body's natural defense mechanisms. The combination of various healing herbs can often enhance their effects. However, care should be taken not to use too many herbs simultaneously. A proven mixture consists, for example, of equal parts thyme, sage, and fennel, which can be brewed as tea and given over the feed.

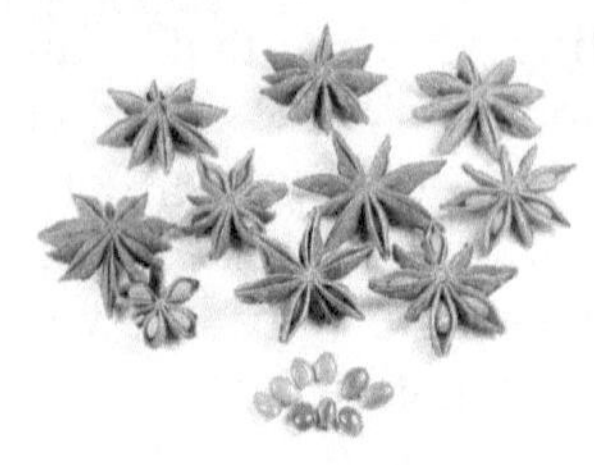

Anis [i29]

Glossary

Bioavailability
The proportion of an active substance that is unchanged and available at the site of action in the body.

Curcumin
A yellow plant pigment derived from the root of the turmeric plant, which possesses anti-inflammatory, antioxidant, and antimicrobial properties.

2. 1. 2. Digestive Herbs

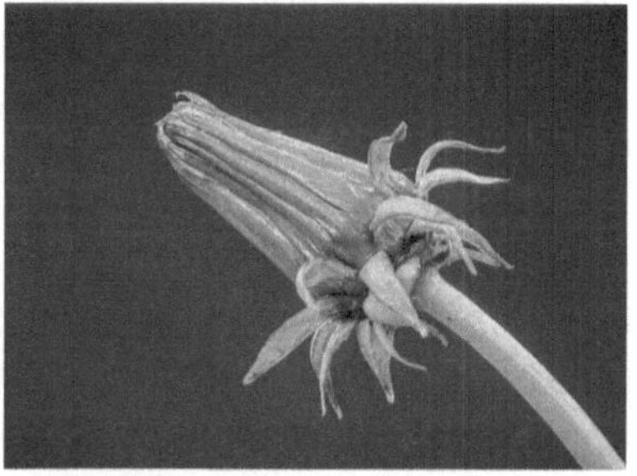

Digestive issues in horses can be effectively treated through the targeted use of medicinal herbs. Traditional herbal medicine offers a wealth of experience that is confirmed and expanded by modern scientific findings [s68]. Dandelion plays a key role in this context. Its digestive-promoting effect is based on several mechanisms: it stimulates bile secretion, supports natural intestinal movements, and optimizes stomach acid production [s68]. In practice, it has proven effective to mix fresh dandelion in small amounts with hay or to add it as dried herb to concentrated feed. It is advisable to start with small quantities and gradually increase the dosage.

Dandelion [i30]

Chamomile is particularly valuable for digestion issues caused by nervousness. Its antispasmodic and calming properties help relieve tension in the gastrointestinal tract [s68]. A practical application is the preparation of a concentrated chamomile infusion, which is added to drinking water. A daily dose of about 15-20 g of dried chamomile flowers is recommended per 100 kg of body weight. An especially interesting aspect is the effect of essential oils on the gut flora. These can specifically reduce pathogenic germs while

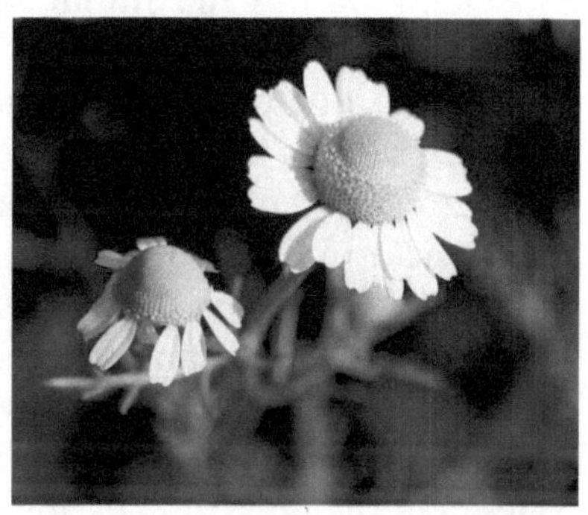

Chamomile [i31]

simultaneously promoting the growth of beneficial gut bacteria [s68]. This property makes them valuable allies in restoring a healthy gut flora, for example, after antibiotic treatments or in cases of digestive disorders.

Alfalfa has proven to be a natural buffer in the digestive tract. Its special properties support the maintenance of a healthy pH level in the stomach and promote fiber digestion [s69]. When feeding, alfalfa should ideally be given before concentrated feed to optimize its buffering effect. The combination of various herbs can enhance their effectiveness. Scientific studies have shown that specially formulated herbal mixtures can improve fiber digestion and positively influence gut health [s68]. A proven mixture consists of equal parts dandelion, chamomile, and

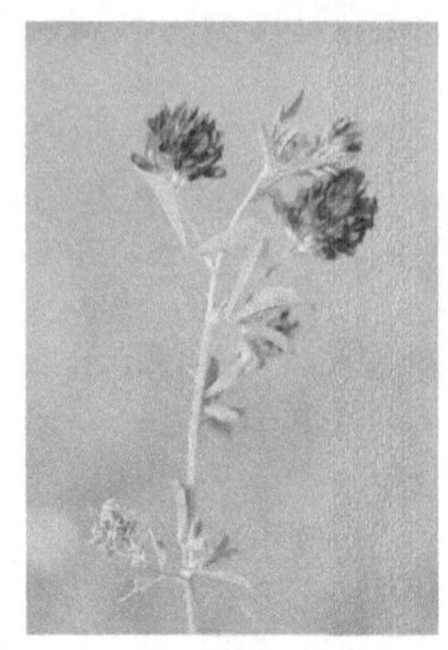

Alfalfa [i32]

alfalfa, which is added to the feed over a period of 2-3 weeks. For practical application, it is important not to combine herbs arbitrarily but to rely on tested mixtures. The dosage should be adjusted to the horse's weight, and treatment for chronic issues should be discussed with a veterinarian. Especially during the initial application, it is advisable to start with small amounts and carefully observe the horse's reaction. The use of herbal powders as dietary supplements has become established in modern horse feeding [s70]. These specially developed products can support the natural gut flora and help with stomach issues. When selecting, one should pay attention to high-quality products specifically designed for horses. A holistic approach to digestive support should consider not only the administration of herbs but also feeding habits and housing conditions. Regular exercise, sufficient roughage, and a low-stress environment are important factors for healthy digestion. The preventive use of digestive herbs can be particularly beneficial in stressful situations such as competitions, transport, or stable changes. Here, the preventive administration of calming and digestive-promoting herbs has proven effective in preventing potential digestive disorders.

Glossary

Alfalfa

A plant from the legume family that can grow up to 1 meter tall and can absorb minerals from deeper soil layers due to its deep root system.

pathogen

Disease-causing or pathogenic - refers to organisms such as bacteria or viruses that can trigger diseases.

2. 1. 3. Immune System Strengthening Plants

he immune system of horses can be effectively supported through targeted herbal administration. Scientific studies confirm the efficacy of various medicinal plants that have been used in traditional medicine for centuries [s71]. Echinacea purpurea (Purple Coneflower) plays a key role in this regard. The plant has been shown to increase the activity of immune cells and improve both cellular and humoral immune defense [s72]. In practical application, it has proven effective to administer Echinacea as a tincture or dried herb prophylactically during the damp and cold season. A daily dose of 15-20 ml tincture or 20-25 g dried herb is recommended per 500 kg body weight.

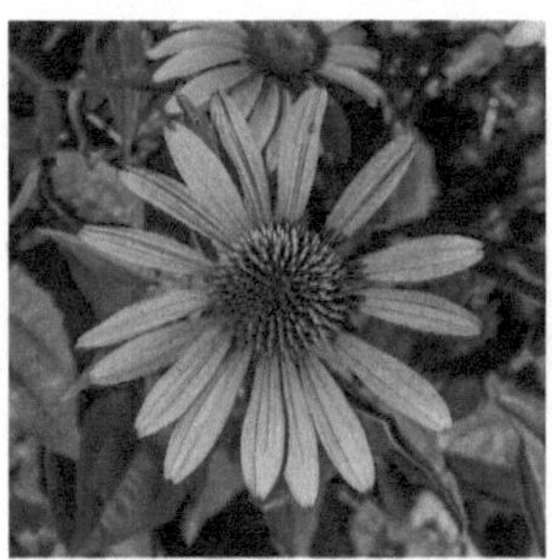

Purple coneflower [i33]

Glycyrrhiza glabra (Licorice Root) exhibits remarkable immunomodulatory properties. It activates macrophages and granulocytes, thereby supporting the body's defense [s73]. When applied, the root should be mixed into the feed as powder or extract. It is important to follow a course of 2-3 weeks with a subsequent break.

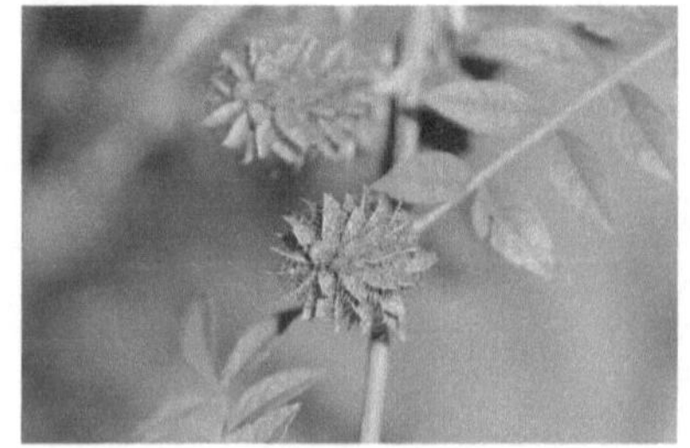

Glycyrrhiza glabra [i34]

Origanum vulgare (Oregano) has proven to be a promising immunomodulator [s72]. Its essential oils have antimicrobial effects and strengthen the immune system. In practice, oregano can be mixed fresh or dried into the feed. A well-established method is also to prepare a concentrated infusion to be added to drinking water.

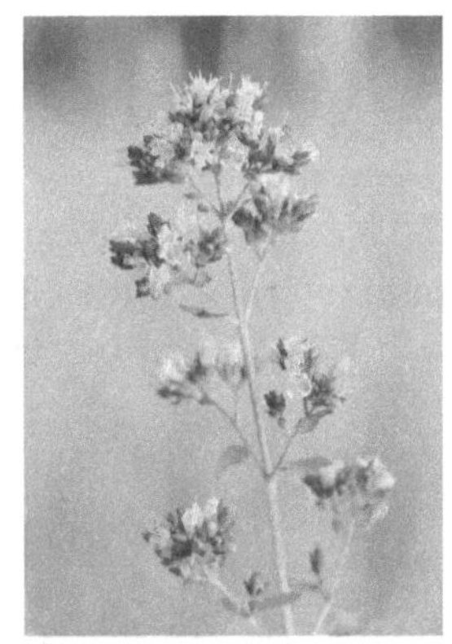

Oregano [i35]

Curcuma longa (Turmeric) and Zingiber officinalis (Ginger) complement each other excellently in their immune-strengthening effects [s71]. While turmeric acts particularly anti-inflammatory, ginger supports the immune system through its metabolism-boosting properties. The combination of both roots can be mixed into the feed as powder, starting with small amounts.

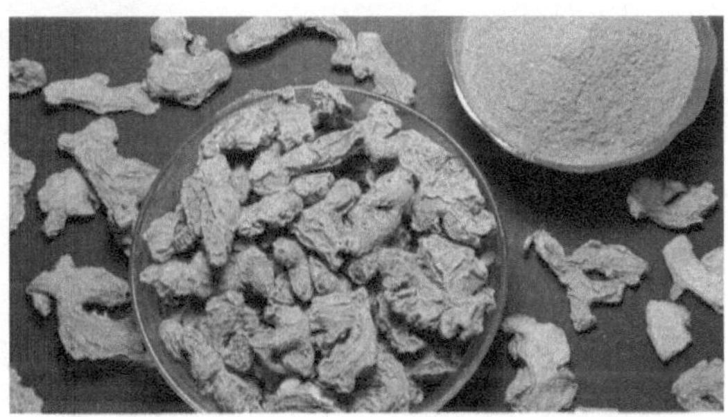

Zingiber officinalis [i36]

Allium sativum (Garlic) has proven to be a natural antibiotic and promotes the production of immunoglobulins [s73]. It is important that the horse accepts the taste during administration. A gentle acclimatization through gradual dose increase has proven effective.

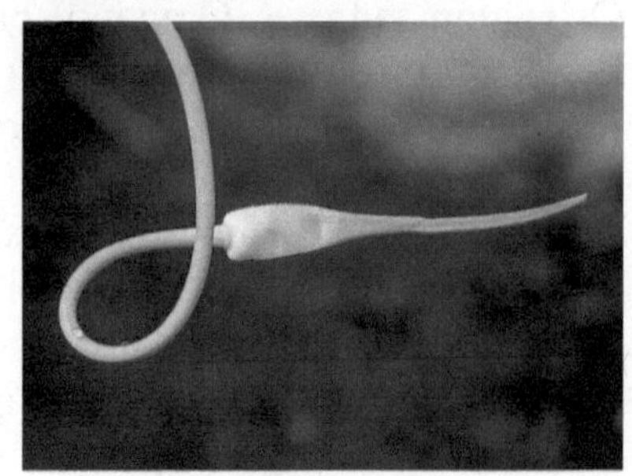

Allium sativum [i37]

<u>Moringa oleifera</u> shows promising properties in supporting the immune system [s71]. The leaves are rich in vitamins and minerals and can be added dried to the feed. Moringa has proven particularly valuable during recovery after illnesses.

When practically applying immune-strengthening plants, some basic rules should be observed:
- The herbs should be administered in courses (2-3 weeks)
- A combination of a maximum of 3-4 herbs is recommended
- The dosage must be adjusted to the horse's weight
- Tolerance should be monitored during the first application
- Chronic diseases require consultation with a veterinarian

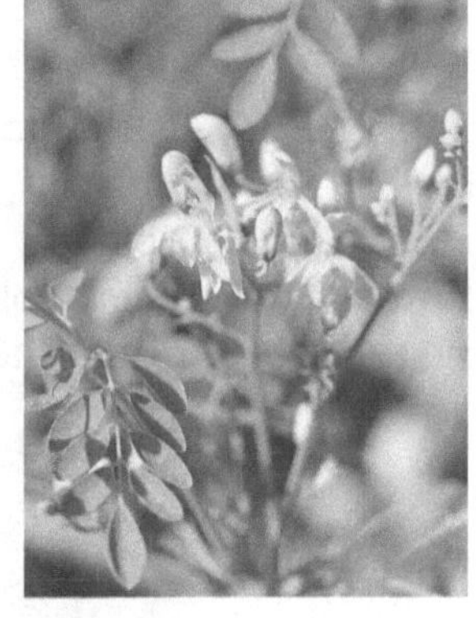

Moringa oleifera [i38]

The preventive application of immune-strengthening herbs is particularly effective in stressful situations such as:
- Competition phases
- Stable changes
- Transport stress
- Weather changes
- Group changes

A well-established basic mixture for immune strengthening consists of:
- 40% Echinacea purpurea
- 30% Origanum vulgare
- 30% Glycyrrhiza glabra

This mixture can be added to the feed over 2-3 weeks, followed by a one-week break. If necessary, the course can be repeated. Research shows that the phytochemicals contained in medicinal plants, such as flavonoids, saponins, and alkaloids, significantly contribute to the immune-strengthening effect [s71]. These substances not only support the direct defense against pathogens but also optimize the body's immune response.

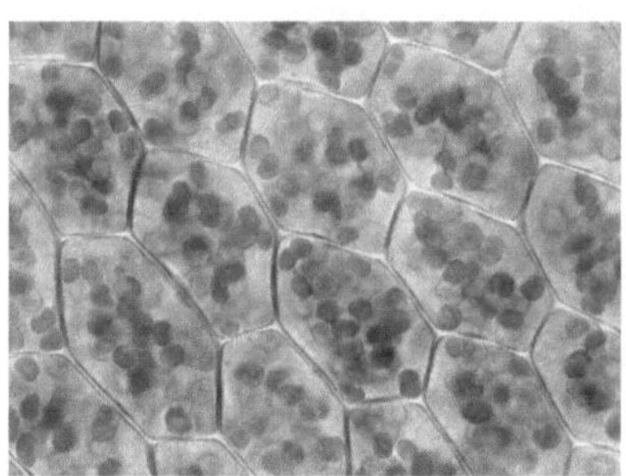

Phytochemikalien [i39]

Glossary

Curcuma longa

A tropical plant from the ginger family with large elongated leaves and yellow flowers, whose rhizome is intensely yellow-orange in color.

Echinacea purpurea

A perennial plant from North America that can grow up to 150 cm tall and features characteristic violet-pink flowers with spiky flower heads.

Glycyrrhiza glabra

A perennial plant that can reach up to 2 meters in height, with feathery leaves and blue to violet flowers, whose roots taste about 50 times sweeter than sugar.

Moringa oleifera

A fast-growing tree from the drumstick tree family that can reach up to 12 meters in height and has tripinnate leaves.

Origanum vulgare

An aromatic member of the mint family with a woody stem, found wild in Europe and Asia, bearing pink to purple flowers.

2. 1. 4. Wound Healing Herbs

Wound healing in horses can be effectively supported through the targeted use of medicinal herbs. Various plants with their specific active ingredients play an important role in the regeneration of injured tissue and the defense against infections [s74].

The marigold (<u>Calendula officinalis</u>) has proven particularly effective due to its wound-healing and anti-inflammatory properties. It can be applied as an ointment or tincture directly to the affected areas. It is important to thoroughly clean the wound beforehand and to carry out the treatment regularly. A practical application method is the preparation of a marigold ointment: Marigold flowers are infused in olive oil and then processed with beeswax to a spreadable consistency [s74].

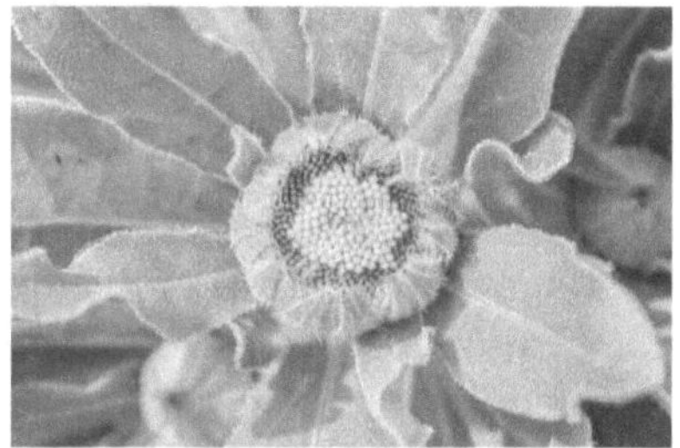

Calendula officinalis [i40]

St. John's wort (<u>Hypericum perforatum</u>) exhibits remarkable properties in wound healing. Its antibacterial and tissue-healing properties make it a valuable aid in the treatment of cuts, abrasions, and postoperative wounds. In practice, the application as an oil extract has proven effective, which is carefully applied to the affected areas [s74]. Myrrh, a traditional remedy, is used in wound treatment due to its <u>antifungal</u> and <u>antiseptic</u> properties. As a diluted tincture, it can be used for wound cleaning and disinfection. The application should initially be tested on a small area to ensure compatibility [s74].

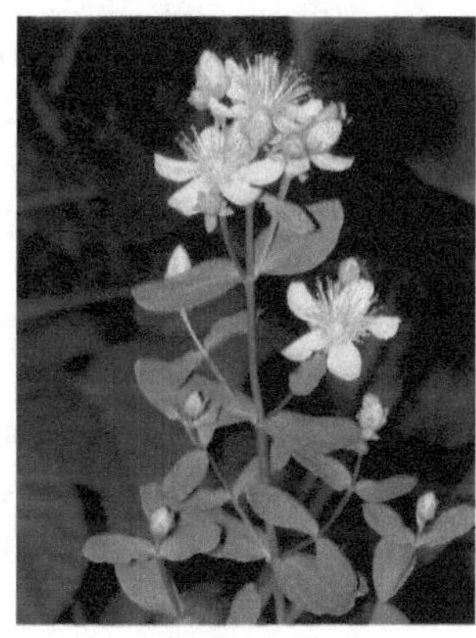

St. John's wort [i41]

A promising approach is the combination of various medicinal plants in the form of wound dressings. Scientific studies have shown that specially developed herbal preparations can accelerate wound healing and reduce the risk of infection [s75]. A proven combination consists of:
- Marigold for tissue regeneration
- St. John's wort for antibacterial action
- Chamomile for anti-inflammatory effects
- Yarrow for hemostasis

When practically applying wound-healing herbs, several important principles should be observed: 1. Thorough wound cleaning before each treatment 2. Sterile application of the preparations 3. Regular monitoring of the healing process 4. Documentation of the treatment 5. Always consult a veterinarian for deep or heavily contaminated wounds

Plantain (<u>Plantago lanceolata</u>) has proven particularly effective for superficial injuries. Its healing-promoting ingredients support the natural regeneration of the skin. In traditional use, fresh leaves are crushed and applied directly to small wounds [s76]. The combination of external treatment with wound-healing herbs and the internal use of immune-boosting plants has proven particularly effective. The herbs used internally support the healing processes from within, while the external treatment acts directly at the site of injury [s75]. For successful wound treatment with medicinal herbs, a systematic approach is important:

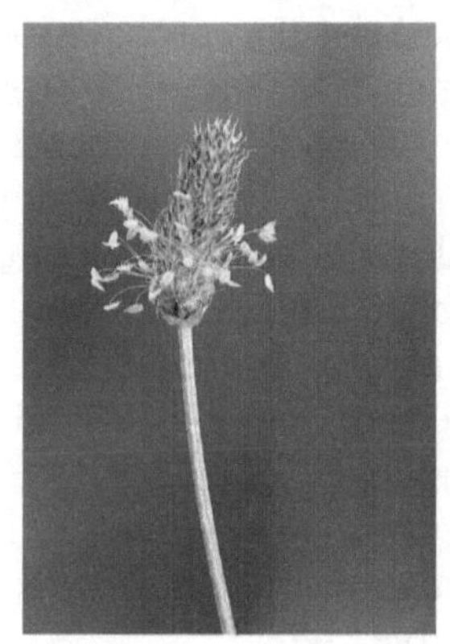

Plantago lanceolata [i42]

1. Phase: Wound cleaning and disinfection
- Thorough cleaning with a diluted herbal tincture
- Removal of dirt and dead tissue

2. Phase: Wound treatment
- Application of the appropriate herbal preparations
- Protection of the wound from external influences

3. Phase: Healing support
- Regular monitoring of the healing process
- Adjustment of treatment as needed

When using wound-healing herbs, it is important to support and not disturb the natural healing processes. The treatment should always be performed with clean hands and sterile materials. In case of signs of complications such as severe swelling, pus formation, or delayed healing, a veterinarian should be consulted immediately.

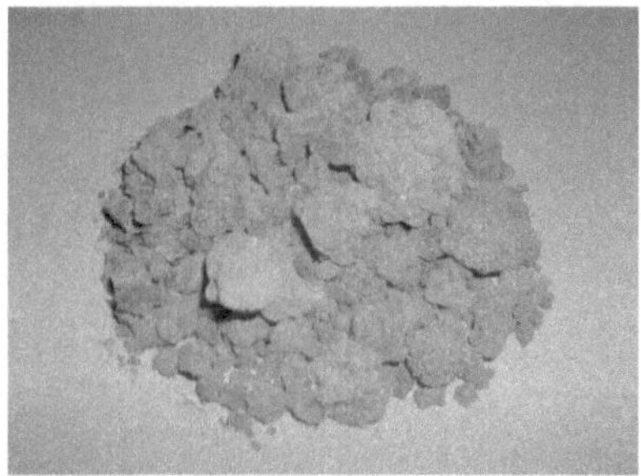

Myrrhe [i43]

Glossary

antifungal
Refers to the property of inhibiting or killing the growth of fungi

antiseptic
Refers to the germicidal or germ-inhibiting effect on
microorganisms such as bacteria and fungi

Calendula officinalis
Latin name of the marigold, which belongs to the family Asteraceae
and originally comes from the Mediterranean region

Hypericum perforatum
Latin name of St. John's wort, a plant indicator of poor soil,
belonging to the family Hypericaceae

Plantago lanceolata
Latin name of plantain, a perennial herb from the family
Plantaginaceae with characteristic lanceolate leaves

Summary - 2. 1. Herbal Medicine

- Thyme contains essential oils with mucolytic and antibacterial properties, with a dosage of 2-3g of dried herb per 100kg of body weight. Water-soluble curcumin has been shown to reduce the production of harmful oxygen compounds in the respiratory tract. Essential oils can specifically reduce pathogenic germs while simultaneously promoting the growth of beneficial gut bacteria. Alfalfa acts as a natural buffer in the digestive tract and should ideally be given before concentrated feed. Echinacea purpurea has been shown to enhance the activity of immune cells and improve both cellular and humoral immune defense. Glycyrrhiza glabra activates macrophages and granulocytes to support the body's own defense. Moringa oleifera shows promising immune-boosting properties and has proven particularly effective during convalescence. A proven basic mixture for immune strengthening consists of 40% Echinacea purpurea, 30% Origanum vulgare, and 30% Glycyrrhiza glabra. Phytochemicals such as flavonoids, saponins, and alkaloids significantly contribute to the immune-boosting effects of medicinal plants. St. John's Wort exhibits antibacterial and tissue-healing properties in the treatment of cuts, abrasions, and postoperative wounds. Myrrh acts antifungally and antiseptically in wound treatment.

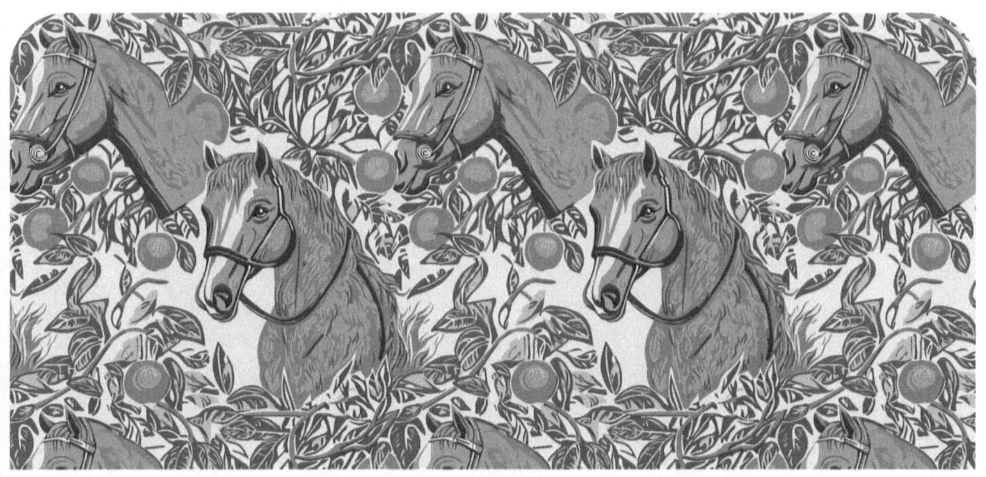

2. 2. Physiotherapy

ow can we optimally support the natural healing processes of the horse's body? What role does physiotherapy play as a holistic treatment approach? These questions concern therapists, veterinarians, and horse owners alike when it comes to the health maintenance and rehabilitation of horses. Physiotherapy for horses encompasses various treatment methods that specifically target the musculoskeletal system, the nervous system, and metabolic processes. From classical manual therapy to innovative taping techniques and specialized forms of massage, it offers a wide range of options to prevent and treat ailments. While some of these methods are based on millennia-old experiential knowledge, modern scientific insights have led to a deeper understanding of their mechanisms. The integration of these insights into practical application now allows for precise and effective treatment of various health issues in horses. The following sections will illuminate the most important physiotherapeutic techniques in detail and demonstrate how they can complement each other to achieve optimal treatment outcomes.

„Manual therapy not only promotes circulation and relieves muscle tension but also supports lymphatic drainage in the horse's body."

2. 2. 1. Manual Therapy

Manual therapy is a central component of the physiotherapeutic treatment of horses and encompasses various techniques performed by trained therapists using their hands [s77]. This form of therapy aims to address movement restrictions and restore the functionality of the musculoskeletal system. A key aspect of manual therapy is massage, which has various positive effects on the horse's body. It promotes circulation, relieves muscle tension, and supports lymphatic drainage [s78]. When performing a massage, it is important to proceed systematically and closely observe the horse's reactions. Therapists typically start with gentle, superficial strokes and gradually increase the pressure according to the individual needs of the horse [s79]. The myofascial release represents a specific form of manual therapy. Here, targeted pressure is applied to the connective tissue (fascia) to release adhesions and improve mobility [s78]. This technique requires a special sensitivity, as the treatment can sometimes be uncomfortable for the horse. Experienced therapists continuously adjust the intensity based on the horse's reactions [s80]. Another important component is targeted stretching exercises. These help restore normal muscle length and prevent stiffness [s78]. Stretches should always be performed slowly and in a controlled manner. A practical example is carefully extending a front leg, holding the leg in position for about 30 seconds to achieve effective stretching of the rear shoulder muscles.

Joint mobilization is another central technique of manual therapy [s81]. This involves performing passive movements of the joints to improve their mobility and optimize joint lubrication [s78]. This technique requires solid anatomical knowledge and should only be performed by trained professionals. The NeuroSomatic Therapy represents an integrative approach that analyzes and corrects structural and biomechanical patterns [s82]. This form of therapy is particularly effective for chronic complaints and takes into account the

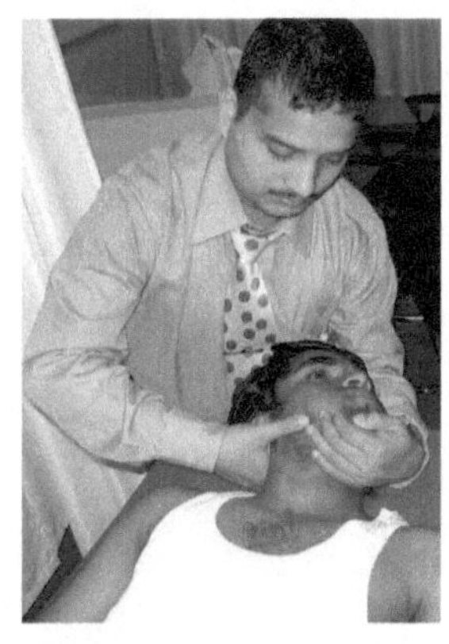

Joint mobilization [i44]

complex interplay of muscles, tendons, and ligaments. Modern physiotherapy centers often combine manual therapy with technological aids such as video motion analysis [s83]. This allows for precise documentation of treatment progress and continuous adjustment of therapy. For the long-term success of treatment, aftercare is of great importance. Therapists often develop individualized exercise programs that horse owners can perform between treatments [s79]. These may consist of simple stretching exercises or controlled movement sequences. The effectiveness of manual therapy is based on various physiological mechanisms. In addition to the direct mechanical effects on tissues and joints, influences on hormone levels, parasympathetic activity, and circulation have also been demonstrated [s77]. This explains the holistic effect of the treatment on the organism. A professional therapist always tailors the treatment to the individual horse, taking into account factors such as age, condition, and any pre-existing conditions [s79]. The duration and intensity of the treatment are modified according to the horse's reactions to achieve optimal results.

Glossary

myofascial

Refers to the treatment of muscles and their surrounding connective tissue layers. The therapy is based on the understanding that these tissue layers form a cohesive network throughout the body.

NeuroSomatic Therapy

A holistic treatment method that utilizes the connection between the nervous system and body structures. It was developed in the 1980s and combines elements from various manual therapy approaches.

parasympathetic

Part of the autonomic nervous system responsible for the body's rest and regeneration. Also referred to as the 'rest nerve,' it promotes digestion and relaxation.

2. 2. 2. Kinesiological Taping

inesiological taping has established itself as an innovative and effective treatment method in equine health. This technique, originally derived from human medicine, utilizes elastic tape strips specifically designed for therapeutic application [s84]. The uniqueness lies in the material's properties, which resemble the thickness and elasticity of the superficial skin layer, allowing optimal interaction with the tissue. In horses, kinesiological taping has a wide range of applications. It is successfully used for tendon and ligament issues, joint dysfunctions, as well as for treating swellings and spinal misalignments [s85]. A practical example is the treatment of a mare with back problems: By strategically applying tape strips along the back muscles, not only was mobility improved, but a significantly more positive overall mood of the horse was also achieved. The mechanism of action of kinesiological taping is based on various principles. The elastic properties of the material create a gentle lifting effect on the skin, influencing the underlying tissue layers [s84]. This micro-manipulation leads to improved blood circulation and supports lymphatic drainage, which is particularly beneficial in cases of swelling and edema. For instance, in a horse with joint swelling, the tape can be applied using a specific lymphatic technique, actively supporting the healing process. Another important aspect is the proprioceptive effect of taping. Through constant gentle stimulation of the skin receptors, the horse's body awareness is enhanced [s85]. This is especially valuable in correcting postural errors or supporting rehabilitation after injuries. For example, in a horse with shoulder issues, targeted taping can optimize muscle activation and positively influence movement patterns. The application of kinesiological taping requires in-depth knowledge and practical experience. Therapists must not only master various taping techniques but also possess a deep understanding of equine anatomy and biomechanics [s86]. In specialized training, they learn the correct application of the tapes, the selection of appropriate techniques, and the assessment of the individual situation of the horse. The versatility of kinesiological taping is particularly noteworthy. It can be used both in the acute phase of an injury and for chronic problems [s84]. The method also combines excellently with other physiotherapeutic techniques. A practical example is the combination of manual therapeutic techniques with supportive taping, often resulting in longer-lasting treatment success. The application always follows a systematic approach: First, a thorough analysis of the issue is conducted, then the appropriate taping technique is selected, and the tape is applied considering the individual anatomy and movement patterns of the horse [s87]. The effect should be continuously monitored to make adjustments if necessary. Another advantage of kinesiological taping is the possibility of extended therapeutic effects between treatment sessions [s84]. Depending on the application and skin compatibility, the tape can remain on the horse for several days, continuously supporting the healing process during this time. This is particularly valuable in treating chronic complaints or during the rehabilitation phase after injuries.

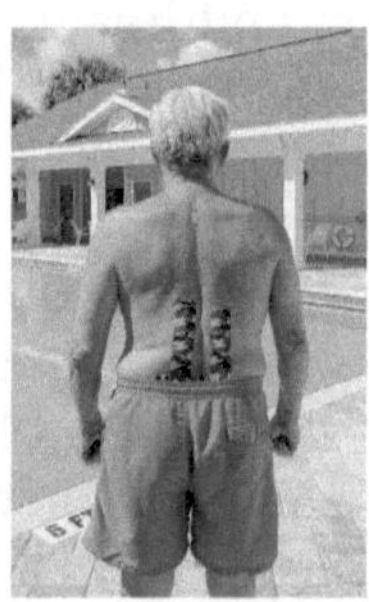

kinesiology taping [i45]

Glossary

Proprioceptive
Refers to the body's self-perception in space through specialized sensory cells in muscles, tendons, and joints. This perception is crucial for balance and coordination.

2. 2. 3. Massage Techniques

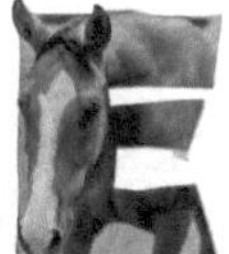quine massage therapy encompasses various specialized techniques that are specifically employed to promote the health and performance of the animal [s88]. Unlike superficial petting, these are systematic treatment methods that require a solid understanding of anatomy.

A central technique is <u>Shiatsu</u>, a form of massage originating from Japan. This involves applying targeted pressure with fingers, hands, elbows, and even knees on specific points along the energy pathways (<u>meridians</u>) [s88]. An experienced therapist can, for instance, relieve blockages in a horse with tense back muscles by systematically working along the bladder meridians. The treatment always begins gently and is adjusted in intensity according to the horse's reactions.

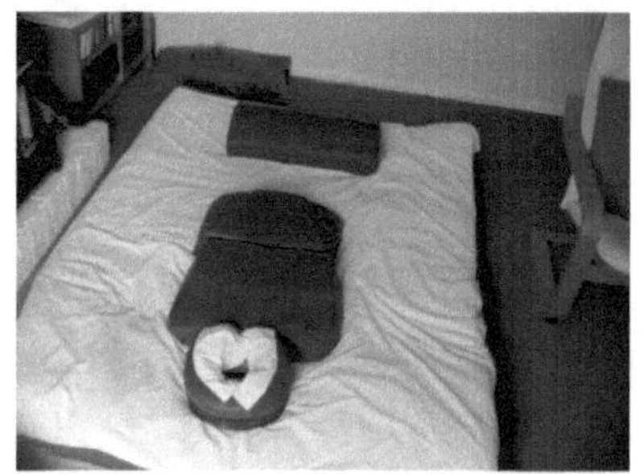

Shiatsu [i46]

<u>Acupressure</u> represents another important massage technique, where pressure is applied to specific body points using the fingertips [s88] [s89]. These points correspond to the acupuncture points known from traditional Chinese medicine. A practical application example is the treatment of the "Bladder 60" point on the hind leg to alleviate tension in the lumbar muscles. The therapist applies gentle, circular pressure for about 30-60 seconds. Particularly in young horses, a combination of various massage techniques has proven beneficial [s90]. Especially during growth phases, regular treatments can help balance unilateral loads and develop better body awareness. A typical treatment protocol might consist of a 15-minute Shiatsu massage followed by targeted acupressure at relevant points. The therapeutic effect of massages is based on various physiological mechanisms [s91]. In addition to the direct mechanical impact on the tissue, energetic aspects are also considered. The treatment aims to release blockages and harmonize the energy flow in the body. This can positively affect the quality of movement and the overall well-being of the horse. For sustainable treatment success, the correct frequency and intensity of massages are crucial [s88]. In acute issues, several treatments per week may be advisable, while monthly sessions are often sufficient for prevention. An

individual treatment plan takes into account factors such as age, type of use, and any pre-existing conditions of the horse. The integration of massage techniques into a holistic therapy concept has proven particularly effective [s90]. Here, massages are combined with targeted conditioning exercises. An example would be massaging the shoulder muscles before practicing stretching exercises to optimize flexibility. The effectiveness of the treatment can be verified through regular documentation of progress. Therapists pay particular attention to changes in muscle tension, movement quality, and the general behavior of the horse. These observations are incorporated into further treatment planning and allow for continuous optimization of the therapy.

Glossary

Acupressure

A healing method where pressure applied to specific body points can alleviate discomfort, based on the same principle as acupuncture, but without needles.

Meridian

Invisible energy pathways in the body that, according to traditional Eastern medicine, transport life energy and connect a network of over 360 points.

Shiatsu

A holistic treatment method from traditional Japanese healing arts, based on the theory of life energy 'Ki', which activates self-healing powers through gentle to deep pressure.

Summary - 2. 2. Physiotherapy

- Manual therapy combines massage, myofascial relaxation, and joint mobilization to restore the functionality of the musculoskeletal system. NeuroSomatic therapy analyzes and corrects structural and biomechanical patterns in chronic complaints. Modern physiotherapy centers utilize video motion analysis for precise documentation of treatment progress. Manual therapy has been shown to influence hormone levels, parasympathetic activity, and circulation. Kinesiological taping employs elastic strips that resemble the thickness and elasticity of the skin layer. Micromanipulation through taping enhances blood circulation and lymphatic drainage through a lifting effect on the skin. The proprioceptive effect of taping optimizes body awareness through constant stimulation of skin receptors. Shiatsu massage systematically works along the meridians with pressure applied by fingers, hands, elbows, and knees. Acupressure targets specific points such as "Bladder 60" for the targeted release of tension. The integration of massage techniques with conditioning exercises demonstrates particular therapeutic effectiveness.

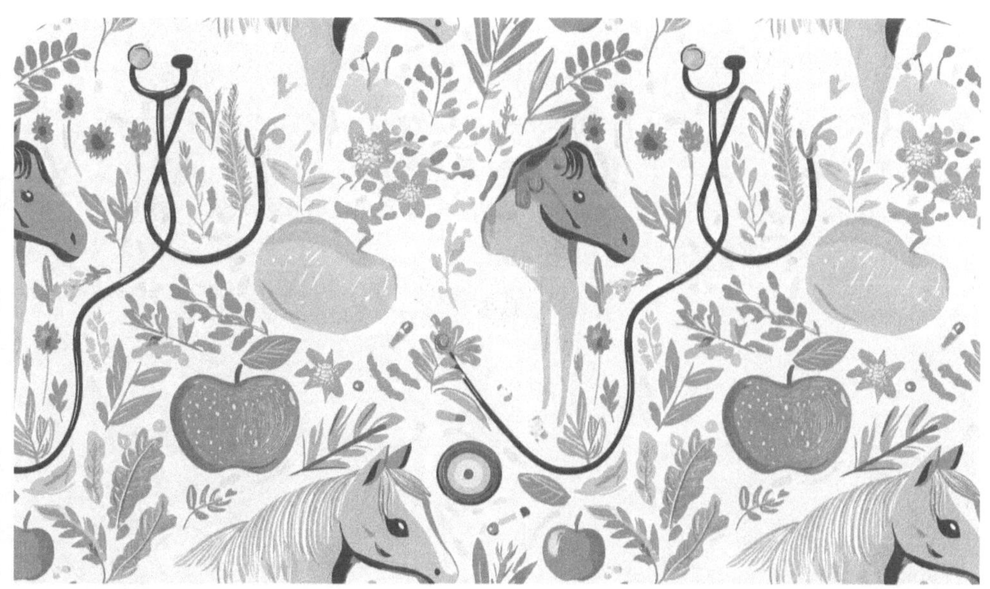

2. 3. Alternative Therapies

he search for effective and compatible therapy forms for horses occupies both veterinarians and horse owners alike. While conventional medicine offers indispensable treatment methods, interest in complementary therapeutic approaches is steadily growing. But which alternative treatment methods have established themselves in equine medicine? How can their effectiveness be scientifically assessed? And what role can they play in the overall concept of horse health? The following sections illuminate four significant alternative therapy forms - acupuncture, osteopathy, homeopathy, and Bach flower therapy. Each of these methods is based on its own theoretical foundations and practical experiences. An objective examination of their possibilities and limitations helps horse owners and therapists make informed decisions for the well-being of their animals.

„Acupuncture has been shown to promote the release of mesenchymal stem cells into the bloodstream, which in turn produce anti-inflammatory proteins and endogenous opioids."

2. 3. 1. Acupuncture

Acupuncture, an ancient healing practice from China, is gaining increasing importance in modern equine medicine [s92]. As part of Traditional Chinese Veterinary Medicine (TCVM), it is based on the concept of Qi - the life energy - and aims to establish a harmonious balance within the organism [s93]. In practical application, very fine needles are placed at specific body points. These acupuncture points are characterized by a particularly high concentration of free nerve endings, arterioles, mast cells, and lymphatic vessels [s93]. Scientific studies have shown that stimulating these points leads to an increased release of endorphins, anti-inflammatory substances, and hormones [s94]. A particularly innovative approach is electroacupuncture, where a weak electrical current is applied between two needles [s92]. This modern variant has been shown to promote the release of mesenchymal stem cells (MSCs) into the bloodstream, which in turn produce anti-inflammatory proteins and endogenous opioids [s95]. The range of applications for acupuncture in horses is remarkably broad. In reproductive medicine, it is successfully used for issues such as anestrus, uterine infections, or reduced libido in stallions [s96]. In the treatment of respiratory diseases, including asthma, acupuncture shows promising results [s97]. It has proven particularly effective for musculoskeletal complaints such as neck stiffness, back pain, and arthritic changes [s92]. A typical treatment session lasts about an hour, during which most horses tolerate the procedure well and relax. In some cases, mild sedation may be helpful [s92]. Generally, at least three sessions are required for treatment success [s92]. An experienced therapist will conduct a thorough $1 examination before treatment begins and identify potential trigger points [s92]. Practical experience shows that acupuncture is particularly effective when used as a complementary therapy to conventional treatment [s98]. For example, it can shorten the healing time of tendon injuries or enhance the effectiveness of classical pain therapies [s93]. In chronic conditions such as arthritis, many horse owners report a significant improvement in their animals' mobility and a reduction in the required pain medications. An important aspect of TCVM is the individual consideration of each horse. According to this concept, each animal has a specific personality associated with the five elements, which must be taken into account when planning treatment [s93]. Based on this, the therapist creates a tailored treatment plan that may include various techniques such as classical needling, electroacupuncture, <u>aquapuncture</u>, or the massage of acupuncture points [s93]. For horse owners, it is important to understand that acupuncture is not a miracle therapy and should not be used as a sole treatment method [s97]. Rather, it achieves its best effect as part of a holistic therapy concept that includes both traditional and modern treatment methods [s98]. The increasing number of specialized centers and qualified therapists [s99] makes this valuable form of therapy accessible to many horse owners today.

Glossary

Anestrus
A phase of sexual inactivity in mares during which no estrus symptoms occur.

Aquapuncture
A variant of acupuncture in which fluids are injected into acupuncture points.

Arteriole
Small arteries with a diameter of 0.04 to 0.1 millimeters that regulate blood flow in the tissues.

Endorphin
Endogenous painkillers, also known as 'happiness hormones,' that enhance well-being.

Mast Cell
Special immune cells that store important signaling molecules and can release them when needed.

Mesenchymal Stem Cell
Special cells in the body that can develop into various tissue types such as bone, cartilage, or muscle tissue.

Qi
A fundamental life energy according to Chinese belief, flowing through invisible pathways (meridians) in the body and regulating its functions.

Trigger Point
Painful knots in the muscles that can cause radiating pain when touched.

2. 3. 2. Osteopathy

Osteopathy represents a holistic manual therapy that views the body as a functional unit and relies on natural healing processes [s100]. This treatment method has proven particularly valuable for horses, as it does not require invasive interventions or additional medications [s101]. The fundamental principles of osteopathic treatment are based on the assumption that all body systems are in close interrelation with one another. The therapist uses their trained hands to palpate and treat dysfunctions in the musculoskeletal system, internal organs, and nervous system. Gentle techniques are employed to activate the body's self-healing powers. A crucial aspect of equine osteopathy is the comprehensive initial examination. The therapist first observes the horse at rest and in motion to identify asymmetries or movement restrictions. This is followed by a systematic palpation

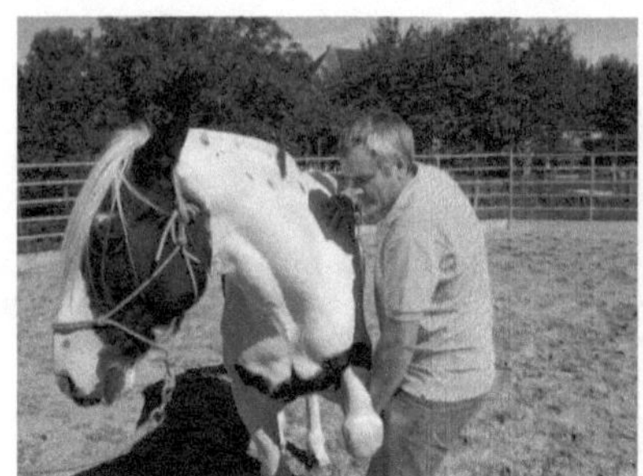

Osteopathy [i47]

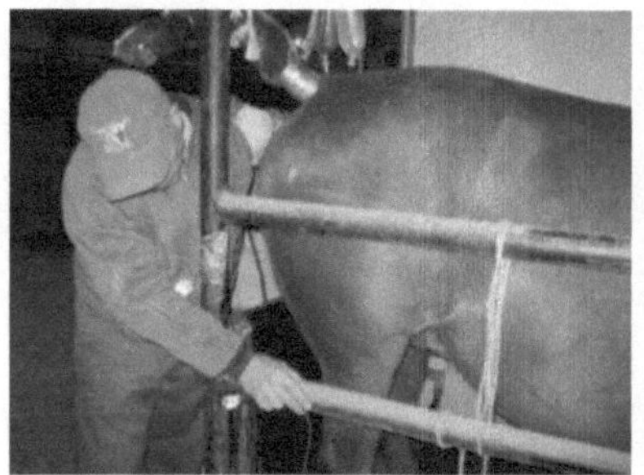

Palpation [i48]

of the entire body. The horse's reaction to specific touches is particularly revealing—pushing away or evading can indicate painful areas. The treatment itself includes various techniques such as gentle mobilizations, rhythmic movements, and specific impulse techniques. An experienced osteopath, for instance, will not only treat the visibly painful region in a horse with back problems but will also search for possible causes in other body areas. Misalignments in the pelvic region, for example, can lead to tension in the back. Scientific studies demonstrate the positive effects of osteopathic treatment. It has been shown that therapy can increase the mechanical nociceptive threshold in horses with and without back pain [s101]. This practically means improved pain tolerance and enhanced mobility. The benefits of osteopathic treatment are manifold. In addition to improving overall health and emotional well-being, treated horses benefit from enhanced joint mobility and optimized recovery after injuries [s102]. Particularly interesting for sport horses is the possibility of increasing performance and minimizing the risk of injury through regular osteopathic treatments. An important aspect of modern equine osteopathy is the integration of Cranial Osteopathy [s102]. This subtle form of treatment addresses the fine movements of the skull bones and their influence on the entire system. This specific technique can be very helpful, especially in cases of head shyness or after dental treatments. For successful treatment, collaboration between the osteopath, veterinarian, and horse owner is essential. The owner should observe some basic behavioral rules after treatment: the horse should not engage in intensive work for 24-48 hours, but light movement is beneficial. Work should also be conducted on soft ground to allow the body to reorganize itself. The professional organization for equine osteopaths, founded in 2013, contributes to the continuous development of this therapy through research and further education [s100]. This ensures high-quality standards and a continuous improvement of treatment methods. It is important for horse owners to know that osteopathy can be used both preventively and therapeutically. Regular check-ups can help identify and address problems early before they manifest. In cases of acute complaints, veterinary clarification is recommended before osteopathic treatment is employed as a complementary therapy.

2. 3. 3. Homeopathy

Homeopathy as a complementary therapy in equine medicine is a subject of controversy. While some therapists and horse owners report positive experiences, veterinary organizations such as the Royal College of Veterinary Surgeons and the British Veterinary Association urge caution in its application [s103]. A central principle of homeopathic treatment is individual therapy. This approach does not primarily focus on the disease symptoms but rather considers the entire appearance of the horse—including behaviors, preferences, and aversions—in the selection of remedies [s104]. This holistic perspective can be particularly significant in treating behavioral disorders. Interesting results are shown in a study on the treatment of stereotypical behaviors in horses. Specific homeopathic remedies were selected according to the individual constitution and the respective behavioral problem. Daily application led to measurable improvements in the animals' behavior [s105]. In practical implementation, it is important for horse owners to administer the remedies regularly and according to a set schedule. Documenting behavioral changes in a therapy diary can be very helpful. A remarkable case report describes the successful treatment of a horse with therapy-resistant wound healing. After unsuccessful conventional treatment of a deep leg wound, alternative therapy led to complete healing within five weeks. Follow-up over a year showed no relapses [s106]. Such case reports can provide important insights for further research but do not replace systematic studies. The scientific evaluation of homeopathy in veterinary medicine is challenging. Numerous randomized controlled trials have so far failed to demonstrate any effect beyond the placebo effect [s103]. This leads to the recommendation that homeopathic treatments should only be used as adjuncts to evidence-based therapies and not as a sole treatment method [s103]. It is important for horse owners and therapists to know that the use of homeopathic remedies should not replace veterinary treatment but only complement it. In cases of acute or severe illnesses, a veterinary diagnosis must always be made first. The decision for or against adjunctive homeopathic treatment should be made in consultation with the treating veterinarian. A growing database of clinical studies and case reports on veterinary homeopathy serves as a resource for further research [s107]. Given global challenges such as increasing antibiotic resistance, there is an urgent need for high-quality scientific investigations to better understand the role of homeopathy in modern equine medicine [s106]. For practical application, a structured approach is recommended: First, a thorough anamnesis should be conducted, which records not only the current complaints but also the horse's temperament, lifestyle, and previous illnesses. The choice of remedies is then made according to the principle of similarity by a qualified therapist. Treatment requires patience but can lead to positive results with consistent implementation [s105].

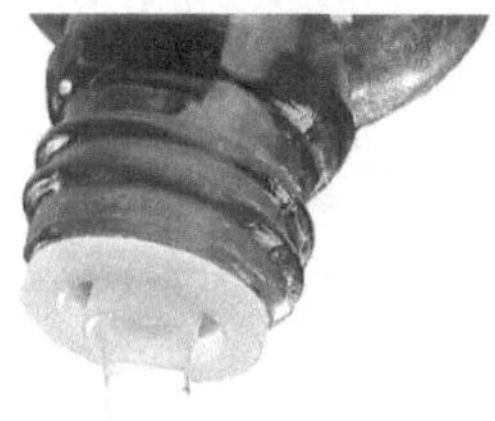

Homeopathy [i49]

2. 3. 4. Bach Flowers

Bach flowers, developed in the 1930s by Dr. Bach, represent a gentle form of alternative therapy that particularly targets the emotional health of horses [s108]. The system is based on 38 different flower essences derived from specific plants, trees, and in some cases, minerals [s109]. These completely non-toxic essences can naturally support the emotional and physical balance of the horse. The fundamental idea of this therapy is based on the <u>holistic</u> approach that physical ailments have an emotional component and should therefore be treated holistically [s110]. This makes Bach flowers a valuable complementary therapy option, especially for behavioral and emotional issues. The range of applications for horses is remarkably broad. Bach flowers have proven particularly effective for:

- Excessive <u>grooming behavior</u>
- Dominance issues within the herd
- Separation anxiety
- Shock states
- Recovery phases after surgeries [s110]

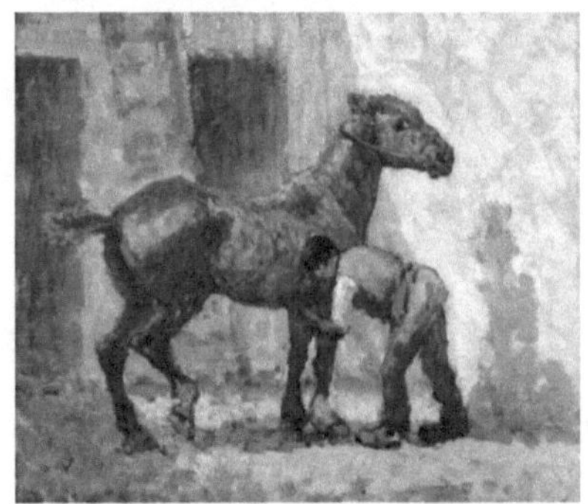

grooming behavior [i50]

The practical application is straightforward. The essences can be administered directly onto the horse's tongue or gums or added to drinking water. The recommended dosage is two to four applications daily [s109]. When used in drinking water, about 10 drops per water container are recommended, with the risk of overdose considered very low [s111]. A unique feature of Bach flower therapy is the possibility of individual composition. Each of the 38 flower essences targets a specific emotional state [s108]. An experienced therapist will create a tailored combination of various essences after a thorough analysis of the horse's character and the issues at hand. The Rescue mixture, a special combination of five flower essences, has proven particularly effective in acute stress situations. It helps restore emotional balance and can be used, for example, before competitions or transport [s109]. Initial effects usually appear after one to two weeks of regular use [s109]. For sustainable results, a treatment duration of at least three months is recommended [s112]. The therapy can be easily combined with other treatment forms [s113], making it a valuable addition to conventional veterinary medicine. Particularly interesting is the use of Bach flowers in preventive health care. They can help to early balance emotional imbalances before they manifest in physical symptoms. This makes them a valuable tool in the holistic health management of horses. The increasing acceptance of this therapy is also reflected in the fact that more and more veterinary clinics and animal welfare organizations are using Bach flowers as a gentle alternative to support animals with emotional problems [s113]. It is especially appreciated that the horse's natural personality remains intact while only undesirable behavior patterns are harmonized.

Glossary

Grooming Behavior
Natural grooming behavior in horses, where they groom and scratch each other or themselves. Serves for coat care and social bonding.

Holistic
Perspective that considers all aspects of a system as a whole rather than analyzing them individually.

Summary - 2. 3. Alternative Therapies

- Acupuncture has been shown to lead to the release of mesenchymal stem cells and endogenous opioids.
- Electroacupuncture enhances the therapeutic effect through weak electrical currents between the needles.
- Acupuncture points exhibit a high concentration of arterioles, mast cells, and lymphatic vessels.
- Osteopathic treatment increases the mechanical nociceptive threshold in horses with back pain.
- Cranial osteopathy addresses subtle movements of the skull bones and their systemic effects.
- A systematic palpation of the entire horse's body allows for the identification of functional disorders.
- Homeopathic treatments have shown success in studies for stereotypical behaviors based on individual constitution.
- Documenting behavioral changes in a therapy diary is essential for homeopathic treatment.
- Bach flower remedies consist of 38 different flower essences and primarily target emotional health.
- The Rescue mixture, made up of five specific flower essences, is successfully used in acute stress situations.
- Excessive grooming behavior can be positively influenced through targeted Bach flower therapy.

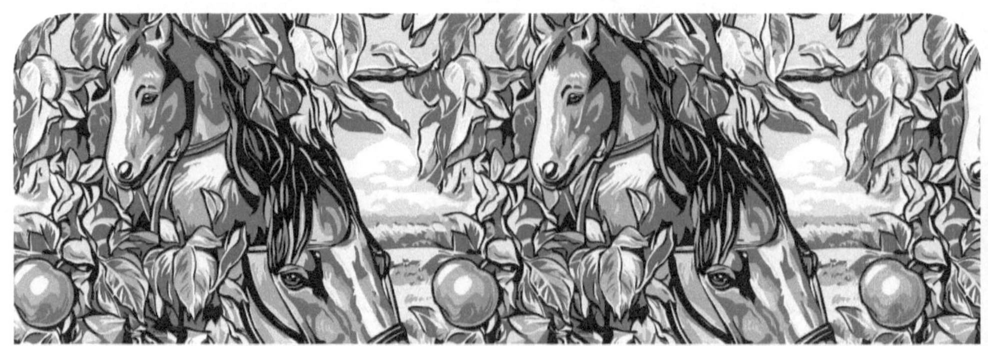

Review - 2. Natural Healing Methods

- Healing herbs such as thyme and eucalyptus are effective for respiratory diseases due to their essential oils.
- Water-soluble curcumin has been shown to reduce the production of harmful oxygen compounds.
- The combination of mint and fennel synergistically supports mucus dissolution.
- Dandelion optimizes stomach acid production and supports natural intestinal movements.
- Alfalfa acts as a natural buffer in the digestive tract and promotes fiber digestion.
- Myofascial relaxation specifically releases adhesions in connective tissue through controlled pressure.
- Electroacupuncture promotes the release of mesenchymal stem cells into the bloodstream.
- Cranial osteopathy addresses the subtle movements of the skull bones and their systemic effects.
- Homeopathic treatments have shown measurable improvements in stereotypical behavior in studies.
- Bach flower remedies have been proven to support emotional balance, especially in stressful situations such as competitions.
- The Rescue mixture of five specific Bach flowers helps to restore emotional balance acutely.
- While these natural healing methods demonstrate impressive successes, a solid medical foundation remains essential—what this should entail will be discussed in the next chapter.

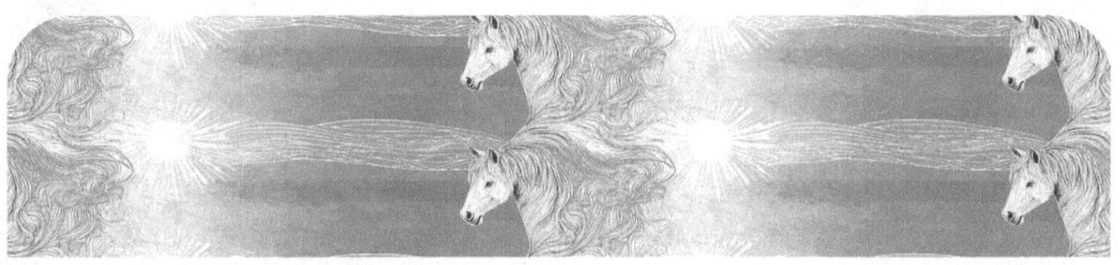

3. Basic Medical Care

he basic medical care of horses requires in-depth knowledge, careful planning, and quick action in emergencies. But what materials should be available in a well-equipped stable pharmacy? How can one recognize the first signs of colic, and what immediate measures should be taken? Regular health care through vaccinations, deworming, and dental checks forms the foundation for a healthy horse life. This raises the question of the optimal frequency of these measures and their correct implementation. Daily hoof care also plays a central role—what aspects should be particularly considered? The following chapters provide essential knowledge for the basic medical care of horses and offer concrete recommendations for emergency situations. Only those who are prepared and know the most important warning signs can react correctly at the crucial moment and provide their horse with the best possible care.

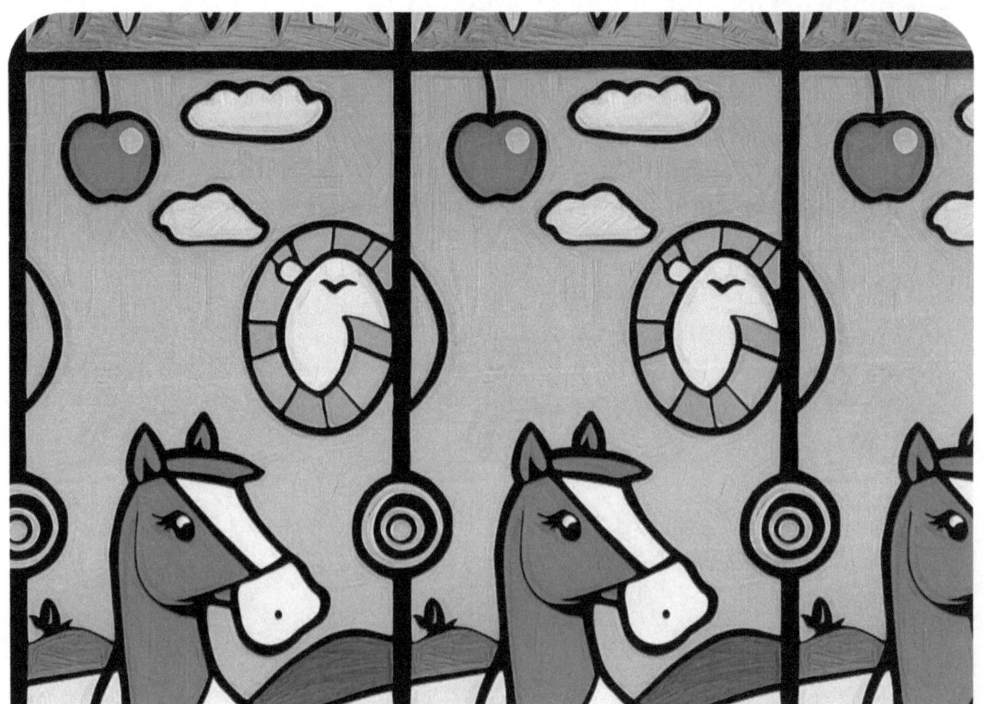

3. 1. Stable Pharmacy

he stable pharmacy is the centerpiece of basic medical care in the horse stable. But what should it really contain? How can the various materials be organized sensibly? And what legal aspects must be considered when storing medications? A well-thought-out stable pharmacy not only enables quick first aid in emergencies but also supports the daily health care of the horses. The systematic organization of bandaging materials, medications, and disinfectants plays a central role in this. Equally important is the regular checking of stock levels and expiration dates. The following sections detail how to professionally set up your stable pharmacy and keep it functional over the long term—so that you are optimally prepared in case of an emergency.

„A well-equipped stable pharmacy is essential for every horse owner, as it enables first aid in emergencies and supports daily health care."

3. 1. 1. Basic Equipment

A well-equipped stable pharmacy is indispensable for every horse owner, as it enables first aid in emergencies and supports daily health care. The basic equipment should be carefully assembled and regularly checked [s114]. Essential components initially include bandaging materials. These consist of elastic and non-elastic bandages in various widths, sterile compresses, cotton wool for dressings, and self-adhesive bandages. These should always be available in sufficient quantities and various sizes. Antiseptic solutions are essential for wound care. It is advisable to have both coloring (e.g., iodine-based) and non-coloring disinfectants on hand, as some injuries require regular wound checks, which could be complicated by discolored skin [s114]. Another important

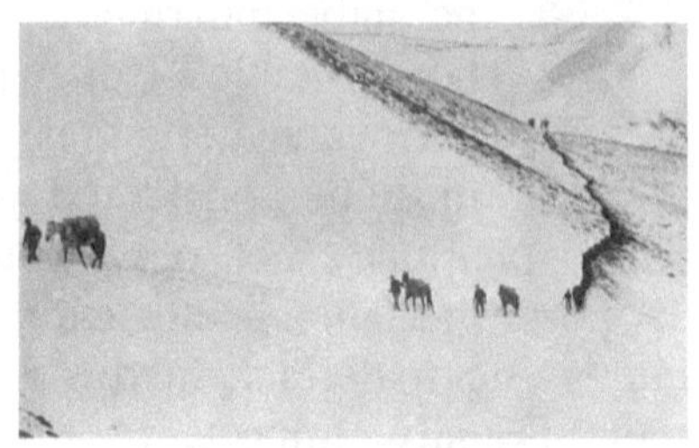

Ice pack [i51]

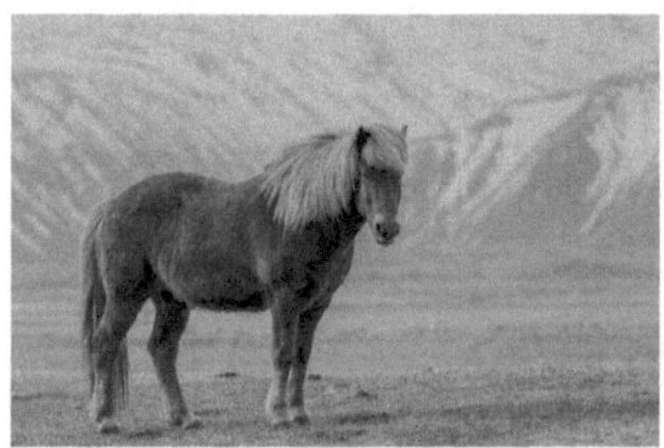

Medications [i52]

aspect is the documentation and organization of emergency contacts. Create a waterproof list of all important phone numbers, especially that of your veterinarian and nearby equine clinics. This list should be prominently displayed in the stable pharmacy. Supplement it with the addresses of the facilities to avoid wasting valuable time searching for this information in an emergency [s115]. For acute injuries, an ice pack is indispensable [s115]. Keep both instant cold compresses and reusable cooling packs on hand. These should be available in various sizes to effectively cool both smaller injuries and larger areas such as joints. The storage of medications requires special care. All medicines should be stored in a lockable, dry, and cool cabinet. Maintain a list of the available medications, their expiration dates, and areas of application. Check this list monthly and replace expired or soon-to-expire medications in a timely manner [s114]. For emergency situations, it is important to have a reserve of basic feed available. Store enough hay for at least three days, as well as a small amount of the usual concentrate feed. Ensure that there is enough water available even in the event of a power outage. A supply of at least 30 liters per horse should always be ready [s114]. Particularly important is the proper storage of all documents. Create a waterproof folder in which you keep copies of all important papers: equine passports, vaccination certificates, current laboratory results, and proof of ownership. Additionally, scan these documents and store them digitally for quick access in an emergency [s114]. Establishing a clear organizational system has proven practical. Divide the stable pharmacy into clearly labeled areas: bandaging materials, medications, cooling, and documents. Label all compartments clearly and create a layout plan so that others can quickly find everything in an emergency. Regular maintenance of the stable pharmacy should occur on a fixed schedule. Create a maintenance calendar and check the inventory, expiration dates, and condition of all materials monthly. Document these checks in writing to keep track and order supplies in a timely manner.

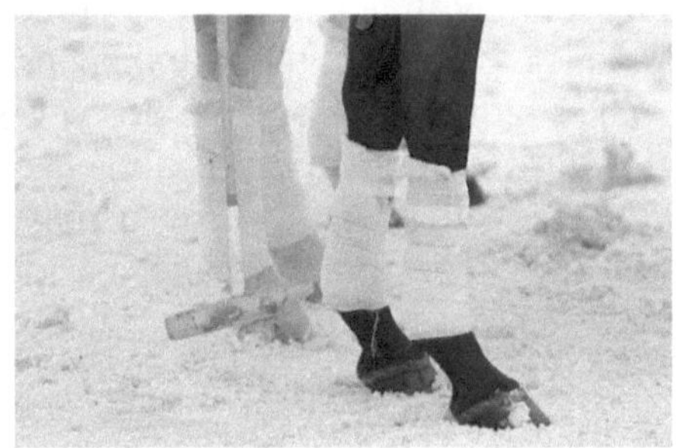

Bandaging materials [i53]

3. 1. 2. Bandaging Materials

Professional wound care for horses requires high-quality and appropriately selected bandaging materials. The correct selection and application of the various materials are crucial for the success of healing. For basic wound care, sterile compresses in various sizes are indispensable. These should be individually packaged to avoid <u>contaminations</u>. When applying, it is important that the compress generously covers the wound edges. A practical rule of thumb is that the compress should extend at least 2-3 cm beyond the wound edges. Padding cotton plays an important role in applying protective bandages. It distributes pressure evenly and prevents the outer bandages from cutting in. Especially for bandages on the limbs, adequate padding is essential. The cotton should be applied in several layers, with each layer secured by a loose fixation bandage. Elastic bandages are another indispensable component of bandaging materials. They allow for a flexible yet stable bandage. The correct tension is crucial during application—bandages that are too tight can impair circulation, while those that are too loose may slip. As a guideline: The bandage should still allow for about a finger's width of indentation.

Self-adhesive bandages have proven particularly effective for securing dressings. They do not stick to the skin or coat but adhere very well to themselves. This allows for a secure hold without additional fastening materials. When applying, the bandage should be wrapped with light tension and overlapping. The frequency of bandage changes depends on the type and condition of the wound [s116]. Heavily oozing wounds require more frequent changes than dry, well-

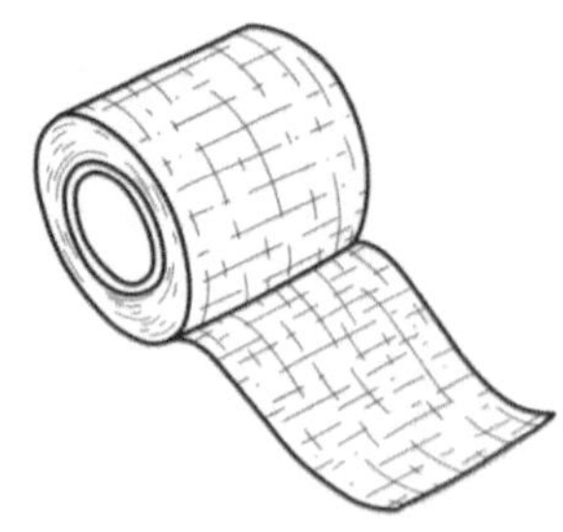

Self-adhesive bandages [i54]

healing injuries. With each bandage change, the wound should be carefully cleaned with $1 solutions [s117]. Sterile swabs or antiseptic wipes are particularly suitable for gentle cleaning. In special cases, plaster casts may also become necessary [s116]. These provide maximum stability and significantly reduce the frequency of bandage changes. However, plaster casts should only be applied under veterinary supervision, ideally with inpatient monitoring of the horse. For the proper storage of bandaging materials, a dry, dust-free cabinet is ideal. All materials should be stored in sealed containers or their original packaging. A systematic arrangement by purpose facilitates quick retrieval in case of need. Regular inventory checks are essential. This should include not only the quantity but also the condition of the materials. Soiled or damaged materials must be sorted out immediately. A guideline for minimum supplies is: At least three complete bandage sets should be available per horse. A practical tip for emergencies: Pack a "first aid bandage kit" in a waterproof box that you can also take on rides. This should be compact yet complete and contain at least compresses, an elastic bandage, and antiseptic wipes. Proper documentation of bandage changes is important for monitoring progress. Record the date, materials used, and observations regarding wound healing. This information is particularly valuable for the treating veterinarian and allows for optimal adjustment of treatment.

Glossary

Contamination

Contamination by pathogens or other harmful substances that can lead to infections during wound care

3. 1. 3. Medications

he proper handling and storage of medications in the stable pharmacy requires special care and responsibility. In principle, medications may only be used and stored in consultation with the attending veterinarian [s118]. This is particularly true for prescription medications. An important component of medication management is the regular deworming of horses. An individual deworming plan should be created, tailored to the parasite load of each horse. The effectiveness of the deworming treatment is verified through regular fecal examinations, which determine the eggs per gram of feces (EPG) [s119]. Deworming for foals begins at the age of two months, although certain active ingredients may only be used from the fifth month of life [s119]. Particular caution is required when using sedatives. These should only be administered by a veterinarian and only when medically necessary [s120]. One should be especially cautious with the administration of medications before travel or transport, as unexpected reactions may occur. A good practice is to document the horse's weight before departure to better assess any potential health changes [s120]. When procuring medications, it is essential to use only regulated and reputable sources [s118]. The use of unapproved or veterinarian-disapproved medications is strictly to be avoided. This also applies to medications that deviate from their licensed use. Veterinarians have the option to choose from a wide range of approved, conditionally approved, or indicated medications [s121]. In certain cases, compressed medications may also be used, but only if they originate from approved products or from the official list of bulk active substances. The use of such preparations should, however, be limited to cases where no other approved treatment options are available [s121].

A practical tip for organizing medications is to maintain a medication log. The following information should be documented:
- Name of the medication
- Batch number
- Expiration date
- Indication
- Dosage
- Date of administration
- Treated horse
- Treatment success

The storage of medications must occur under the conditions specified by the manufacturer. Many preparations require a cool and dark environment. A lockable medication cabinet with an integrated cooling area has proven effective in practice. Regular checks of expiration dates and the immediate disposal of expired medications are essential. In the treatment of respiratory diseases, the choice of the right antibiotic has proven crucial for treatment success [s122]. The decision for a specific preparation should always be based on the experience of the attending veterinarian and, if possible, on an <u>antibiogram</u>.

Glossary

Antibiogram
A laboratory test to determine the sensitivity of bacteria to various antibiotics in order to identify the most effective treatment

Bulk Active Substance
Raw materials for medications in larger quantities used by pharmacies to produce individual medications

Compressed
Specially processed and compacted medications that allow for better handling or dosing

EPG
Unit of measurement for determining worm infestation, assessed through microscopic examination of feces and serving as the basis for the deworming strategy

3. 1. 4. Disinfectants

isinfectants play a central role in the stable pharmacy and are essential for maintaining the health of horses. The correct selection and application of these agents is crucial for their effectiveness [s123]. In general, different types of disinfectants are distinguished, which should be selected according to the area of application and requirements. Phenolic disinfectants have proven particularly effective, as they remain effective even in the presence of organic material such as manure or bedding [s124]. This is especially important, as many pathogens such as <u>rotaviruses</u> or <u>salmonella</u> can survive in organic material [s125]. For daily stable hygiene and during disease outbreaks, a systematic approach is required. The four essential steps are: 1. Thorough removal of all organic material 2. Cleaning with soap and thorough rinsing with water 3. Complete drying of surfaces 4. Application of the disinfectant, observing the prescribed exposure time [s126] When handling disinfectants, correct dosing is crucial. Each agent must be diluted and applied according to the manufacturer's instructions. A concentration that is too low can impair effectiveness, while a concentration that is too high can be harmful to health [s127]. In the event of an outbreak, special hygiene measures are necessary. Infected horses must be isolated, and all contact surfaces must be disinfected. Separate tools such as brooms, shovels, and forks should be used for infected areas [s128]. For hand hygiene between horse contacts, <u>iodophors</u> or alcohol-based hand disinfectants are particularly suitable [s128]. Equipment requires special attention. Bridles, halters, and other equipment must be regularly cleaned and disinfected. The following procedure has proven effective: first, thorough mechanical cleaning, then wiping with a suitable disinfectant cloth or spraying with disinfectant, followed by drying with a clean cloth [s127].

When selecting a disinfectant, various factors should be considered:
- Spectrum of action against specific pathogens
- Compatibility with the materials to be disinfected
- Biodegradability
- Cost-effectiveness [s125]

For the stable pharmacy, it is advisable to keep various disinfectants on hand:
- A phenolic preparation for general stable disinfection
- An iodophor for hand disinfection and instrument cleaning
- An alcohol-based hand disinfectant for quick interim disinfection

Proper storage of disinfectants should be in a separate, lockable cabinet, away from medications and bandaging materials. All containers must be clearly labeled, and the original label with application instructions must be retained [s127].

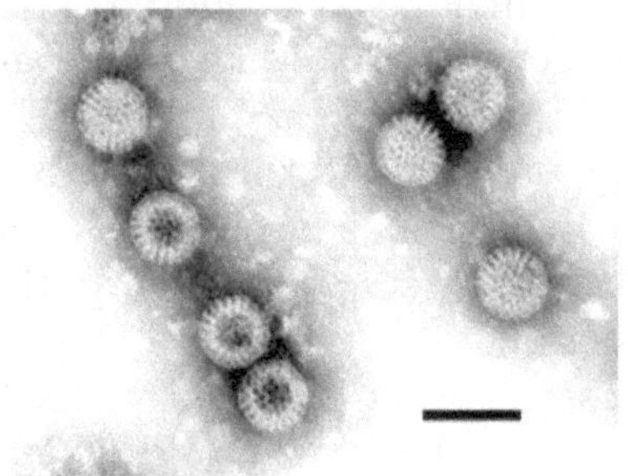

Rotaviren [i55]

Glossary

Iodophor

A special form of disinfectant that contains iodine in a stable
compound with a carrier molecule. It characteristically turns brown
and has a particularly long duration of action.

Rotavirus

A group of viruses that can cause severe diarrhea in young foals.
They are very resilient and can survive in the environment for
several months.

Salmonella

Bacteria that can cause severe gastrointestinal diseases in horses.
They are particularly dangerous as they can also be transmitted to
humans and can spread quickly in the stable.

Summary - 3. 1. Stable Pharmacy

- The stable pharmacy requires at least three complete bandage sets per horse. Phenolic disinfectants remain effective even when in contact with organic material such as bedding. Deworming in foals begins at two months of age; certain active ingredients are only approved from the fifth month of life. Compacted medications may only originate from approved products or the official bulk active substance list. Sterile compresses should extend 2-3 cm beyond the wound edges. The effectiveness of the deworming treatment is monitored by determining EPG (eggs per gram of feces). A water supply of at least 30 liters per horse should always be available. Iodophors are particularly suitable for hand disinfection between horse contacts. The bandage tension should be chosen so that the bandage can still be pressed in about one finger's width. In the event of disease outbreaks, separate tools such as brooms and pitchforks must be used for infected areas.

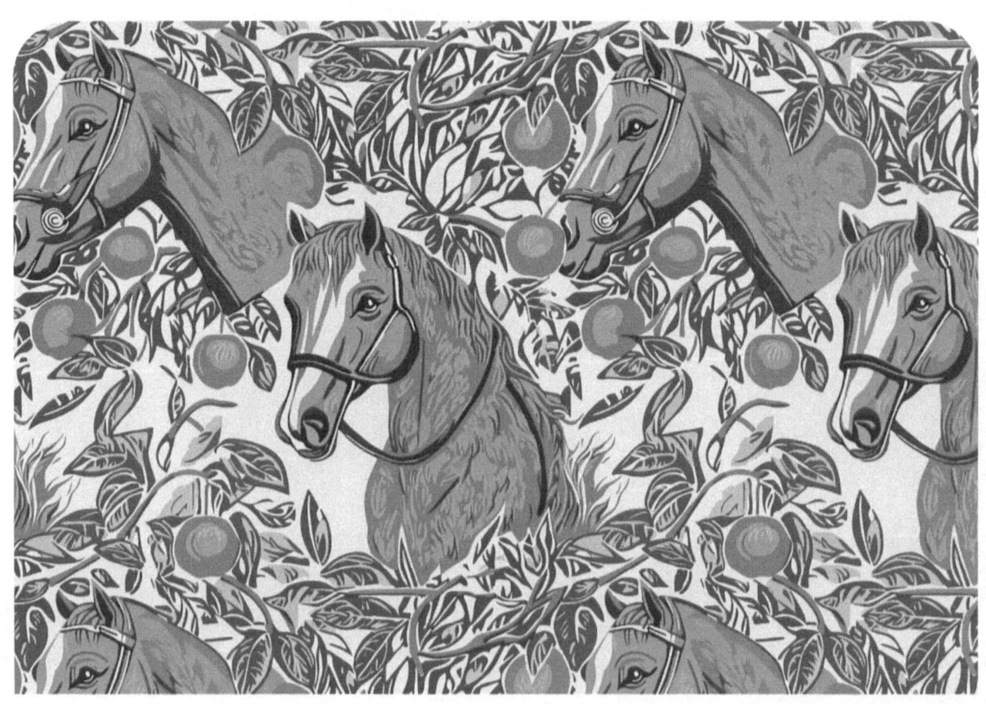

3. 2. First Aid

n critical situations, minutes often determine the health or even the life of a horse. But how can a horse owner recognize the seriousness of the situation? When is swift action required, and when might hasty intervention worsen the situation? First aid for horses requires both solid knowledge and the ability to act thoughtfully in stressful situations. From proper wound care to early recognition of colic signs and life-saving emergency measures—the right preparation and understanding of fundamental principles can be crucial. This chapter imparts essential knowledge for horse owners to respond competently in emergencies while also recognizing their own limits. The measures presented are based on current veterinary medical findings and have been prepared for practical application.

„When initially treating a wound, one should place fresh material on a bleeding dressing without removing the old one, in order to avoid destroying newly formed blood clots."

3. 2. 1. Wound Care

The prompt and knowledgeable care of wounds is particularly important for horses, as these animals are inherently prone to injuries [s129]. The severity of a wound can be deceptive—large, heavily bleeding injuries often appear more dramatic than they are, while small wounds near joints or tendons can be more serious [s130]. In the initial care of a wound, it is essential to remain calm and reassure the horse [s131]. If possible, the animal should be moved to a clean, dry stable or a quiet area. A feed bucket can help distract the horse and keep it calm. It is advisable to involve a second person for support before beginning the wound assessment or first aid. Wound healing occurs in several phases: inflammation, <u>cell migration</u>, tissue deposition, and skin contraction [s132]. To enable optimal healing, wounds should ideally be sutured within six hours [s132]. The following procedure should be observed during initial care: 1. For bleeding wounds, apply even pressure with a sterile, absorbent bandage. Important: If the bandage becomes soaked, place fresh material on top without removing the old one to avoid disrupting newly formed blood clots [s129]. 2. After controlling the bleeding, assess the wound in terms of location, depth, and severity. A 0.9% saline solution is suitable for cleaning [s132]. Tap water can also be used, but caution is advised for wounds near joints or tendons [s132]. 3. For heavily contaminated wounds, an antimicrobial wash solution containing iodine may be used [s133]. The water stream should not be too strong to avoid pushing contaminants deeper into the wound [s131].

A veterinarian should be consulted immediately in cases of:
- Severe bleeding
- Wounds that penetrate the full thickness of the skin
- Injuries near joints or tendons
- Visible deeper structures
- Heavily contaminated wounds [s130]

Until the veterinarian arrives, no pain relief should be administered, as this may complicate the assessment of the wound [s129]. The use of topical medications should also be avoided initially [s132]. A proper wound dressing consists of three layers: 1. Primary layer: direct contact with the wound 2. Secondary layer: padding 3. Tertiary layer: fixation and compression [s129]

Every horse owner should have a well-equipped first aid kit for wound care.
This should include:
- Sterile wound dressings
- Antiseptic solutions
- Bandages
- Clean bucket
- Scissors
- Thermometer
- Large towels
- Current phone number of the veterinarian [s130]

A particular challenge in wound healing can be the formation of excessive
granulation tissue (also known as "proud flesh") [s133]. This can hinder
healing and requires veterinary treatment. Proper wound care can help
prevent this complication. Further wound treatment should be conducted in
close consultation with the veterinarian [s134]. For small wounds, it is
advisable to change the dressing every 2-3 days, while monitoring for signs
of infection [s130]. An up-to-date tetanus vaccination is essential for all
horses, as even small, unnoticed wounds can lead to dangerous infections
[s133].

Glossary

Cell Migration
   Directed movement of cells in the tissue, where healing cells
   actively move towards the wound to support the healing process.

Granulation Tissue
   Newly formed connective tissue during wound healing, consisting
   of small reddish elevations and important for healing. However,
   excessive formation can become problematic.

3. 2. 2. Colic Signs

olic in horses is a medical emergency that requires prompt action. Symptoms typically develop in varying degrees of severity and must be recognized early to avoid serious consequences [s135]. Even in mild cases, horses exhibit initial characteristic signs: they curl their lips, intensely observe their flanks, and become restless. They often begin to paw the ground with their hooves [s135] [s136]. As a horse owner, you should be particularly attentive during this phase and closely monitor your horse's behavior. Lead the horse for a maximum of 10 minutes to see if the symptoms improve [s135]. In moderate colic cases, symptoms become significantly more pronounced. The animals frequently urinate, lie down repeatedly, and stand back up. A characteristic sign is also prolonged lying on their side [s135]. During this phase, it is important to keep the horse away from hard or sharp objects that could cause injury when lying down. Document the frequency and duration of the symptoms—this information is valuable for the veterinarian. Severe colic cases manifest through intense rolling, heavy sweating, and rapid breathing. The animals can sustain injuries to their body and face due to uncontrolled rolling and thrashing [s135]. At this stage, immediate veterinary assistance is essential. Until the veterinarian arrives, you should try to prevent further injuries and monitor the vital signs. An important indicator of the severity of colic is the eating and drinking behavior. Affected horses often show complete disinterest in food and water [s137]. Sweating often occurs in characteristic patterns (patches). Continuous monitoring of vital signs, especially heart rate and temperature, provides important insights into the animal's stress state [s137]. Particular attention is required in cases where a <u>diaphragmatic hernia</u> may be the cause. Symptoms can vary widely and depend on which organs are affected [s138]. In large defects, the large intestine may become trapped, leading to recurrent colic. A characteristic feature is the simultaneous occurrence of colic and respiratory distress symptoms [s138]. Certain laboratory values can be helpful for differential diagnosis. In equine grass sickness (EGS), for example, the levels of <u>serum amyloid A</u> and <u>fibrinogen</u> are elevated, distinguishing them from non-inflammatory colic causes [s139]. These findings assist the veterinarian in targeted diagnosis and treatment.

As a horse owner, you should contact a veterinarian immediately in the following situations:
- If symptoms persist for more than 30 minutes
- In case of a significant deterioration in condition
- If severe symptoms such as intense rolling occur
- If respiratory problems occur simultaneously
- If the horse does not consume food and water for an extended period

Accurate observation and documentation of symptoms, as well as timely recognition of severity, are crucial for successful treatment. Ideally, create a schedule in which you note the observed symptoms and their intensity. This information is extremely valuable for the attending veterinarian.

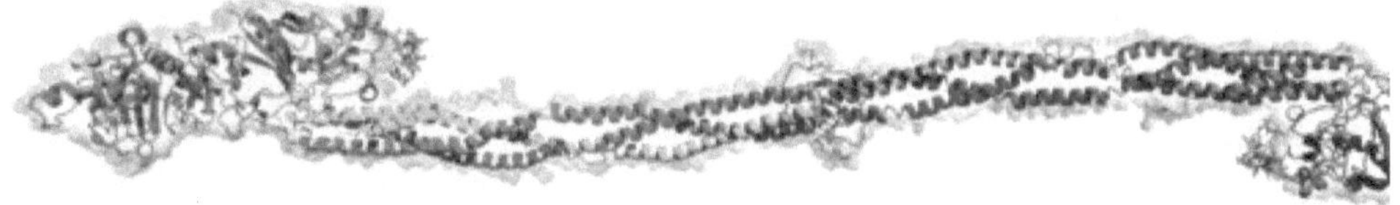

Fibrinogen [i56]

Glossary

Diaphragmatic Hernia

A tear or defect in the diaphragm that allows organs from the abdominal cavity to move into the thoracic cavity. Can be congenital or caused by injuries.

Fibrinogen

A protein produced in the liver that is important for blood clotting and increases during inflammation in the body. It is used as a diagnostic marker.

Serum Amyloid A

A protein produced during inflammation in the body that serves as an important inflammatory marker in the blood. It is classified as an acute-phase protein.

3. 2. 3. Emergency Measures

n emergency situations, swift and deliberate action is crucial for the health and survival of the horse. A well-thought-out emergency plan and proper preparation form the foundation for successful crisis management [s140]. In principle, all individuals who regularly handle the horse should be trained in basic first aid. This particularly includes recognizing signs of stress such as behavioral changes, loss of appetite, and physical symptoms like increased sweating or rapid breathing [s141] [s142].

When preparing for emergencies, creating a comprehensive emergency plan is essential. This should include the following elements:
- Current contact information for veterinarians and transporters
- Documentation of all important health information
- Permanent identification of the horses (microchip/tattoo)
- Current vaccination and health documentation
- Emergency supplies for 48-72 hours [s140]

A particularly critical emergency is heatstroke. If body temperatures exceed 40.5°C, immediate action is required. The horse should be promptly moved to the shade and cooled with water at room temperature, focusing particularly on areas with large blood vessels. Good air circulation is essential. While access to fresh water must be ensured, the horse should not be forced to drink [s143] [s144]. In the case of severe injuries, the principle is to move the horse as little as possible unless it is absolutely necessary for safety reasons. Foreign objects in wounds should never be removed independently, as this can lead to increased bleeding. This task should be left to a professional in a controlled environment [s141] [s144].

In the event of a necessary evacuation, a priority list should be created. This includes:
- Three-day supply of hay, feed, and water
- Important documents
- First aid kit
- Ropes and halters
- Water buckets
- Identification halter
- Contact and accommodation lists [s145]

Another critical emergency is the risk of choking. In this case: Immediately remove food and water and promptly seek veterinary assistance. Attempts to resolve an obstruction on your own can worsen the situation and should be avoided [s142]. For a horse that is down, it is important not to force the animal to stand up. Instead, a veterinarian should be contacted immediately. Until their arrival, the horse should be kept warm and dry [s142].

The first aid kit should be regularly checked and replenished. Essential components include:
- Medical tape
- Gauze sponges
- Bandage scissors
- Disposable gloves
- Thermometer
- Emergency flashlight
- <u>Tourniquet</u> (only for arterial bleeding) [s144]

When applying a tourniquet, extreme caution is required. It must be loosened every five minutes to ensure blood circulation in the remaining limb [s144]. The emergency plan should be practiced regularly to ensure routine action in case of an emergency. It is always paramount that the safety of people takes absolute priority, followed by the safety of the horses [s140] [s145].

Glossary

Tourniquet

A medical constriction system for controlled interruption of blood flow. It typically consists of a wide band with a fastening mechanism and is used only in life-threatening bleeding situations.

Summary - 3. 2. First Aid

- Wounds should ideally be sutured within six hours for optimal healing.
- For bleeding dressings, place new material over the old rather than removing it to protect blood clots.
- Wound healing progresses through the phases of inflammation, cell migration, tissue deposition, and skin contraction.
- Excessive granulation tissue ("proud flesh") can hinder healing.
- In colic, horses exhibit characteristic sweating patterns in the form of patches.
- Serum amyloid A and fibrinogen levels are elevated in equine grass sickness.
- Diaphragmatic hernias can lead to recurrent colic and simultaneously show symptoms of respiratory distress.
- In heatstroke with temperatures above 40.5°C, cooling must be concentrated on areas with large blood vessels.
- A tourniquet must be loosened every five minutes to ensure blood flow.
- The emergency supply should be designed for 48-72 hours.

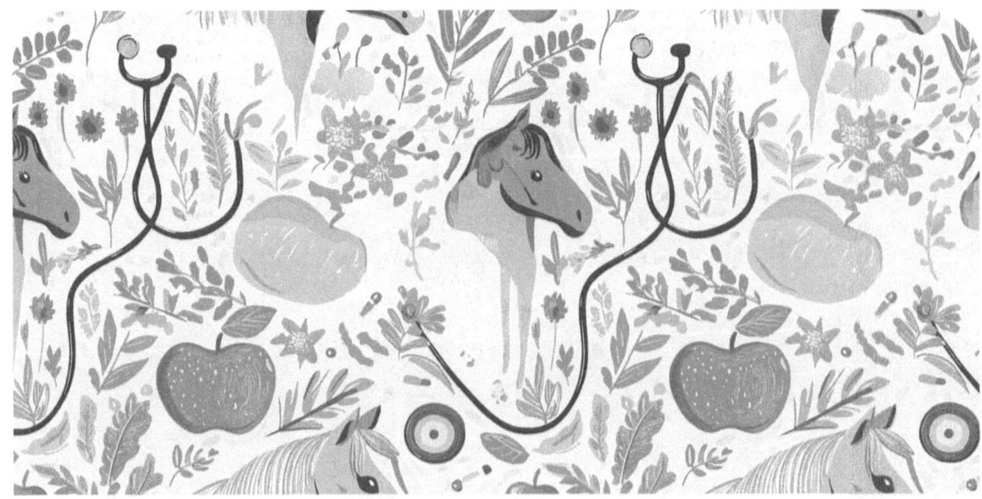

3. 3. Preventive Examinations

egular medical check-ups form the foundation for the long-term health maintenance of horses. But which examinations are truly necessary? How often should they be conducted? And what role do the horse's age and usage type play in this? From dental checks to vaccinations, systematic worm control, and professional hoof care—each area of preventive care follows its own principles and requires specific expertise. The challenge lies in integrating these various aspects into a coherent overall concept. Scientific knowledge in equine medicine is continually evolving, leading to new recommendations for preventive health care. A solid understanding of the key preventive measures enables horse owners to make informed decisions regarding the health of their animals.

„About 20% of the horses in a herd carry 80% of the total parasite load.“

3. 3. 1. Dental Check

egular dental checks are an essential component of equine health and should never be neglected. Dental care begins with a first examination shortly after birth for newborn foals to identify potential misalignments or other issues early on [s146]. This early intervention can prevent complicated treatments later. The frequency of dental checks is based on the horse's age: after the initial examination, further checks should occur at three months of age, followed by semi-annual examinations until the fifth year of life [s147]. For healthy adult horses between 6 and 10 years, an annual check is sufficient, provided there are no particular abnormalities [s146]. From the tenth year onward, experts recommend semi-annual examinations again, unless the dentition is in exceptionally good condition [s146]. A professional dental examination begins with taking the medical history. The veterinarian inquires about dietary habits, living conditions, and the horse's overall performance [s148]. Owners should pay particular attention to behavioral changes while eating or riding with a bit, as these can be important indicators of dental problems [s149]. Before the actual dental examination, the horse's vital signs are checked. This includes heart rate, respiratory rate, temperature, and the hydration status [s148]. For a thorough examination, the horse is usually lightly sedated, which minimizes stress for the animal and allows for safe treatment [s150]. Using modern technology, such as high-resolution cameras, the veterinarian can conduct a detailed examination and documentation of the teeth and soft tissues in the mouth [s147]. Special attention is paid to irregular wear, cavities, tooth fractures, and possible infections [s148]. Sharp tooth edges, which arise from the typical grinding motion during chewing, are often identified. One of the most common treatments is known as "floating" - the smoothing of these sharp edges [s146]. This routine treatment is important because sharp tooth edges can lead to injuries of the oral mucosa and cause pain while chewing. A well-functioning dentition is essential for optimal feed utilization and, consequently, for the overall health of the horse [s149]. Malocclusions (misalignments of the teeth) can not only lead to problems with feed intake but can also cause behavioral issues while riding [s149]. The earlier such problems are detected, the better the treatment options. Delaying treatment can lead to increased discomfort or even tooth loss [s149]. After the examination, the owner receives a detailed report on the condition of their horse's teeth and any treatment recommendations [s147]. This documentation is important for tracking dental health and assists in planning future treatments. Regular dental checks are not only important for oral health but can also uncover other health issues [s149]. Investing in dental health pays off through better feed utilization, reduced feed costs, and improved overall health of the horse [s149]. Owners should take the recommended check-up intervals seriously and engage an experienced veterinarian for the examination [s148].

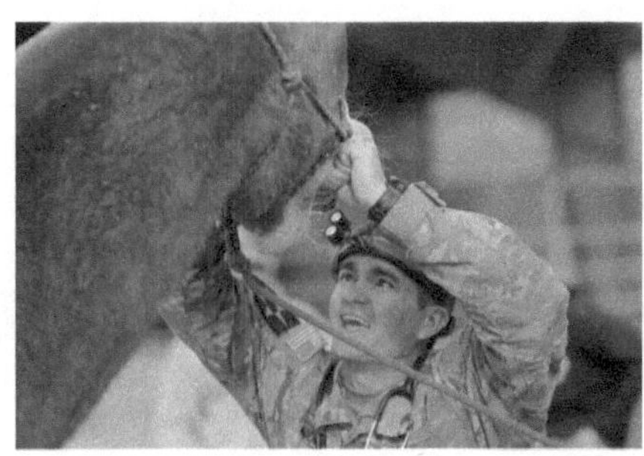

Floating [i57]

Glossary

Floating

A specific dental treatment technique for horses, where special rasps are used to smooth the chewing surfaces of the molars. The term comes from the English 'to float' (to hover/smooth).

Hydration Status

The body's fluid balance, which can be assessed based on various characteristics such as skin elasticity and mucous membrane condition.

Malocclusion

A dental misalignment where the teeth of the upper and lower jaws do not meet correctly. This can be congenital or develop due to uneven tooth wear.

3. 3. 2. Vaccination Prophylaxis

accination prophylaxis is a fundamental component of health care for horses and serves to protect against dangerous infectious diseases [s151]. Unlike other preventive measures, vaccination prophylaxis follows an individually tailored schedule based on the horse's age, its intended use, and specific risk factors. In general, a distinction is made between core and risk-based vaccinations [s151]. Core vaccinations form the foundation of immunization and are essential for all horses, regardless of their use. Owners should note that this basic immunization begins in foals and must be consistently continued. The administration of vaccinations is carried out according to strict protocols established by experienced veterinarians [s152]. It is important to understand that not every vaccine can be administered by anyone—certain vaccinations are prescription-only and must be performed by a licensed veterinarian. Horse owners are advised to maintain a detailed vaccination schedule and to keep vaccination records carefully. Particularly horses that frequently come into contact with other horses, such as at competitions or in stables with high turnover, require more comprehensive vaccination protection. For these animals, a semi-annual vaccination schedule for certain diseases is recommended [s151]. A practical example: a competition horse should be protected not only against core vaccinations but also against specific risk diseases that can be transmitted at equestrian events. The development of modern vaccines and research into immunization strategies is continuously advancing [s153]. This allows for ongoing improvements in vaccine efficacy and optimization of vaccination protocols. Horse owners should regularly consult their veterinarians about new developments and recommendations. An important aspect of vaccination prophylaxis is the documentation of possible vaccination reactions [s152]. Should adverse side effects occur, they must be carefully documented and reported to the attending veterinarian. This helps in adjusting future vaccination strategies and contributes to improving vaccine safety. Veterinary education places great emphasis on understanding the <u>immunological</u> foundations and the correct application of vaccination protocols [s154]. This ensures that veterinarians can optimally advise and treat their patients. Horse owners benefit from this expertise through informed guidance in creating individual vaccination plans. Effective vaccination management requires close collaboration between the veterinarian and the horse owner [s151]. Regular health checks should be combined with the review of vaccination status. A practical tip: many horse owners use digital calendar systems or apps to avoid missing vaccination appointments. Vaccination prophylaxis is important not only for the individual horse but also serves to protect the entire horse population [s155]. Consistent vaccination programs can prevent or at least contain disease outbreaks. This is particularly significant in stable communities, where pathogens can spread rapidly.

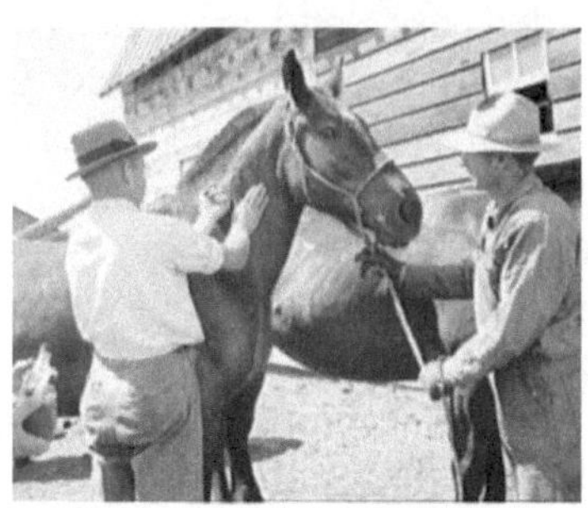

Vaccination prophylaxis [i58]

Immunology

The science that deals with the body's defense mechanisms against pathogens. It examines how the immune system produces antibodies and responds to foreign substances.

3. 3. 3. Deworming

he modern deworming treatment for horses has fundamentally changed in recent years. The previously common practice of routinely treating all horses every six weeks with rotating dewormers is now considered outdated [s156]. Instead, a strategic, individualized approach based on scientific research is increasingly being adopted. Central to this new approach is the regular performance of fecal examinations, specifically the Fecal Egg Count (FEC). These tests should be conducted at least twice a year, ideally in spring and autumn [s157]. They allow for the classification of horses into different categories: low shedders (<200 EPG), moderate shedders (200-500 EPG), and high shedders (>500 EPG) [s158]. Based on this classification, an individualized treatment plan is created. Low shedders require only two treatments per year—in spring (March) and autumn (October). Moderate shedders receive an additional treatment in late summer (July), while high shedders need four treatments per year—in March, June, September, and November [s158]. Particular attention is given to the treatment of foals, which follow a specific protocol. The first deworming occurs at two months of age, followed by regular treatments. From the fourth to fifth month of life, FEC tests should also be conducted for foals [s158]. A practical example: A foal receives its first deworming at two months, the second at four months, and the third at six months, with special attention to strongyles from the fifth month onward [s159]. An important aspect of modern worm management is the assessment of treatment effectiveness. The Fecal Egg Reduction Count Test (FERCT) is used for this purpose [s156]. This test helps to identify resistant worm populations early and adjust the treatment protocol accordingly. A concrete example from practice: If the FERCT shows insufficient reduction in egg count after treatment, the attending veterinarian must change the dewormer. Interestingly, about 20% of the horses in a herd carry 80% of the total parasite burden [s159]. This finding underscores the importance of individualized treatment plans. A practical tip for stable operators: Maintain detailed documentation of FEC results and treatments for each horse to identify trends and optimally adjust the treatment strategy. The American Association of Equine Practitioners recommends that adult horses over three years of age do not need to be routinely dewormed until the fecal egg count reaches at least 200 to 500 EPG [s160]. Nevertheless, every adult horse should receive at least one basic treatment annually that targets both roundworms and tapeworms [s161]. An often overlooked but important aspect is the accurate weight determination of the horse before deworming to avoid underdosing [s160]. A practical recommendation: Use a weight tape or a formula for weight estimation when a scale is not available. The overarching goal of a modern worm control program is not the complete eradication of all parasites—this would be neither realistic nor desirable. Rather, it is about maintaining the health of the horses and minimizing the risk of clinical diseases [s162]. A balanced approach between parasite control and the avoidance of resistance development is key to success.

Glossary

Fecal Egg Count

A laboratory diagnostic method for the quantitative determination of worm eggs in fecal samples. The sample is prepared with a special solution and evaluated under a microscope.

Fecal Egg Reduction Count Test

A specialized laboratory test that assesses the effectiveness of dewormers by comparing the number of worm eggs before and after treatment. The test should be conducted 10-14 days after deworming.

Strongyles

A family of roundworms that are among the most common internal parasites in horses. They can embed in the intestinal wall and lead to colic in cases of severe infestation.

3. 3. 4. Hoof Care

egular and proper hoof care is fundamental for the health and well-being of a horse [s163]. It encompasses various aspects, from daily basic care to professional treatment by a farrier. The foundation consists of daily inspection and cleaning of the hooves [s164]. The hooves should be thoroughly scraped out and examined for signs of problems such as cracks, infections, or other abnormalities. A practical tip for horse owners: integrate hoof cleaning into the daily routine, preferably before and after riding. Pay particular attention to foreign objects like stones or debris that may have lodged in the hoof. Professional hoof treatment by a qualified farrier should occur at regular intervals [s165]. The rhythm depends on various factors such as hoof growth, type of use, and housing conditions. A concrete example: for a normally used riding horse, a 6-8 week shoeing interval is usually appropriate, while sport horses often require shorter intervals.

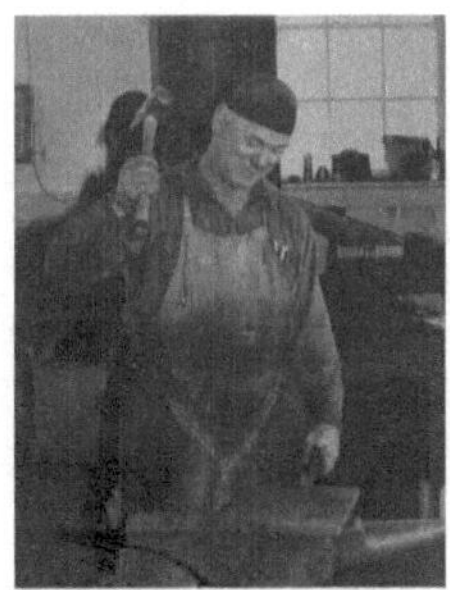

Farrier [i59]

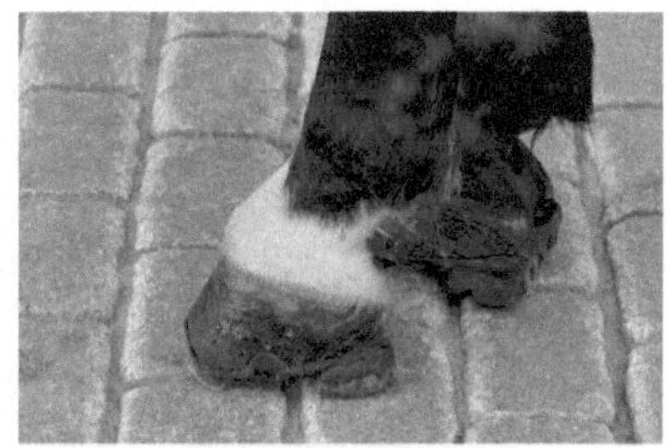

Horseshoe [i60]

The decision between shoes and barefoot should be made individually [s166]. Horseshoes provide additional protection and can be beneficial when indicated. The selection of the right shoeing is crucial and should be tailored to the specific needs of the horse. A practical example: a dressage horse may require a different shoeing than a show jumping horse or a leisure horse.

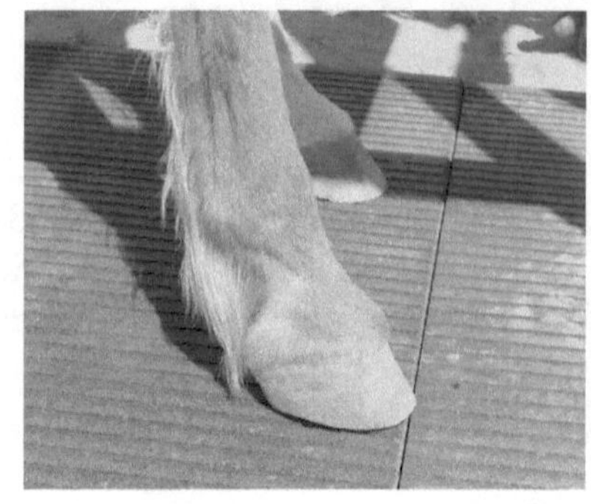

Hoof health [i61]

Various factors significantly influence hoof health [s165]. These include:
- Genetic predisposition
- Nutritional status
- Environmental conditions
- Movement management
- Age of the horse

A holistic care approach considers all these aspects [s167]. It is important to create an individual care plan that addresses the specific needs of each horse. A practical piece of advice: keep a hoof care diary in which you document observations, treatments, and shoeing cycles. The prevention of hoof problems plays a central role [s168]. Regular and correct trimming is essential to maintain the natural hoof shape and avoid misalignments. An important practical tip: pay special attention to hoof hygiene during wet periods, as the risk of thrush and other moisture-related issues increases. Horse owners have various educational opportunities in the field of hoof care [s169]. These range from basic workshops to detailed training on hoof anatomy and care techniques. A practical note: take advantage of these offerings to deepen your knowledge and recognize problems early. The economic significance of good hoof care should not be underestimated [s168]. Neglected hoof problems can lead to significant follow-up costs due to treatments and performance losses. A practical example: regular investment in qualified hoof care is significantly cheaper than treating chronic laminitis or other serious hoof diseases.

Summary - 3. 3. Preventive Examinations

- Dental checks for foals begin immediately after birth and are repeated at three months of age.
- For healthy horses aged 6-10 years, an annual check is sufficient; thereafter, semi-annual examinations are recommended.
- Modern dental examinations utilize high-resolution cameras for detailed documentation.
- 'Floating' refers to the professional smoothing of sharp tooth edges.
- Core vaccinations form the foundation of immunization and begin in foal age.
- Competition horses require a semi-annual vaccination schedule for certain diseases.
- 20% of horses in a herd carry 80% of the total parasite load.
- The fecal egg count (FEC) classifies horses into low (<200 EPG), moderate (200-500 EPG), and high shedders (>500 EPG).
- The Fecal Egg Reduction Count Test (FERCT) assesses the effectiveness of deworming treatments.
- Foals receive their first deworming at two months, followed by additional treatments at four and six months.
- The American Association of Equine Practitioners recommends deworming only at 200-500 EPG for adult horses.
- The shoeing interval for normally used riding horses is 6-8 weeks.
- Sport horses often require shorter intervals between hoof care.

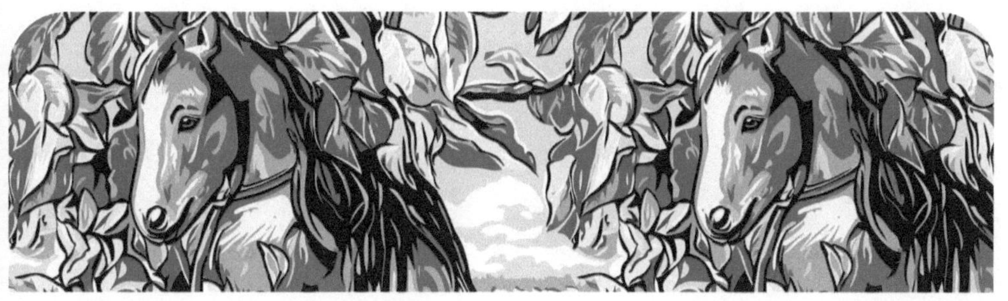

Review - 3. Basic Medical Care

- A well-equipped stable pharmacy includes, in addition to bandaging materials, both coloring and non-coloring disinfectants for optimal wound control. Instant cold compresses and reusable cooling packs in various sizes are essential for the initial treatment of injuries. Medications must be stored in a lockable, dry, and cool cabinet and checked for expiration dates monthly. Phenolic disinfectants remain effective even in the presence of organic material such as feces or bedding. The previously common practice of routine deworming every six weeks is now considered outdated; instead, individualized treatment is based on fecal examinations. Approximately 20% of horses in a herd carry 80% of the total parasite load. The first dental examination occurs in newborn foals, followed by further examinations at three months of age and semi-annual checks until the fifth year of life. Malocclusions can lead not only to problems with feed intake but also to behavioral issues while riding. In vaccination prophylaxis, a distinction is made between core and risk-based vaccinations, with competition horses requiring a semi-annual vaccination schedule. Hoof care by a qualified farrier is performed at shorter intervals for sport horses than for normally used riding horses. While basic medical care forms the foundation for the horse's health, training physiology plays a crucial role in achieving optimal performance.

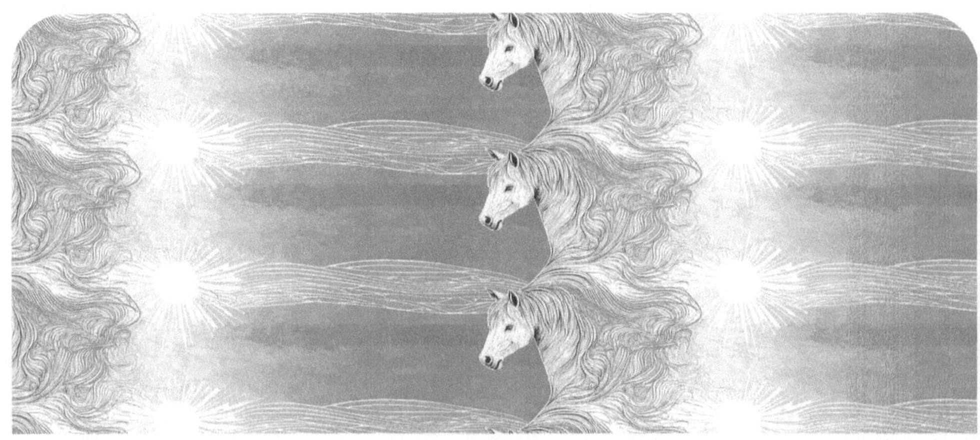

4. Training Physiology

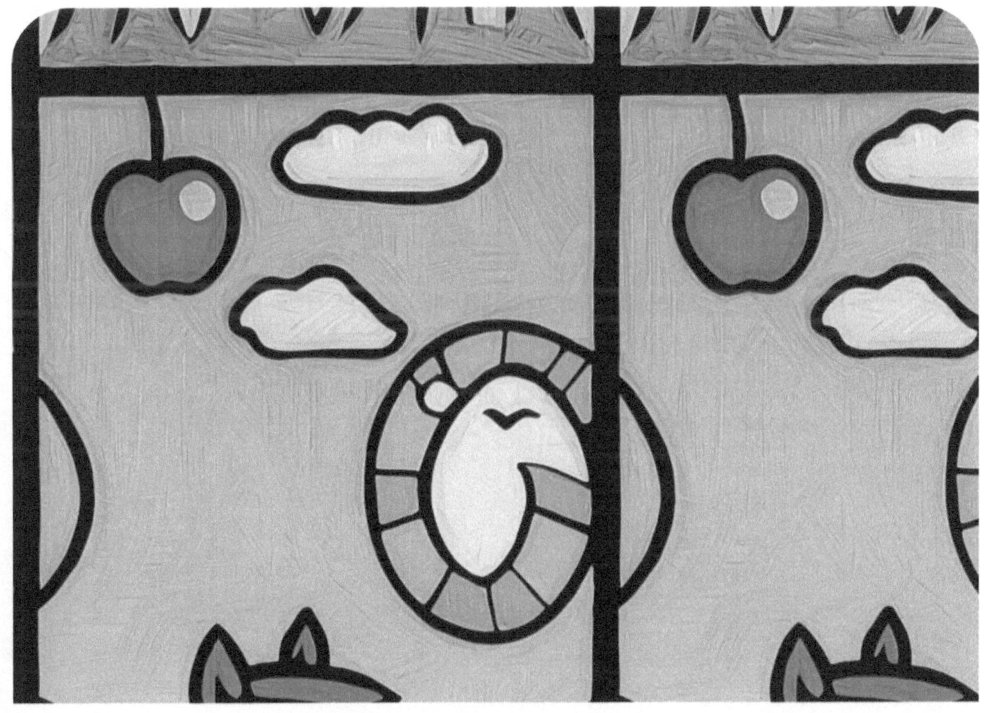

raining physiology forms the scientific foundation for the systematic development and maintenance of horses' health. How can the enormous adaptability of the equine organism be optimally utilized? What role do the various body systems and their complex interplay play in this? From targeted muscle development to the coordination of movement patterns and balance—understanding the underlying physiological processes enables precise training management while considering the individual needs of the horse. Which training stimuli lead to the desired adaptations? How can overexertion be avoided? Modern training physiology combines traditional knowledge with the latest scientific findings. It provides the basis for systematic training planning and effective injury prevention. The following chapters illuminate the various aspects of training physiology and demonstrate how this knowledge can be profitably applied in practical work with horses.

4. 1. Muscle Building

How does muscle tissue develop in horses and what factors influence muscle growth? What role do training, nutrition, and recovery play in this process? These questions concern both horse owners and trainers, as a healthy and well-developed muscular system is the foundation for the horse's performance and health. Muscle development in horses is a complex physiological process that encompasses far more than just regular training. It is based on the interplay of various biological mechanisms—from protein synthesis to hormonal regulation. Understanding these fundamentals allows for the optimal coordination of training methods and recovery phases. Current research continually provides new insights into the molecular processes involved in muscle development and opens up innovative approaches for effective training concepts. These scientific foundations form the basis for systematic and sustainable muscle development in horses.

> *„For muscle building, 2-5 sets per exercise with 5-15 repetitions are optimal.“*

4. 1. 1. Training Basics

A systematic training structure forms the foundation for successful muscle building. It is essential to start with a clearly defined <u>SMART</u> goal—one that is specific, measurable, achievable, relevant, and time-bound [s170]. This could mean, for example, increasing the weight in squats by 20 kilograms within three months. Strength training, also referred to as resistance training, is the central training method where muscles work against an external resistance [s171]. This resistance can take various forms—from body weight to dumbbells to resistance bands. For beginners, a full-body workout performed 2-3 times a week is recommended [s170]. A practical example of a training plan could look like this: full-body training on Monday and Thursday, with an optional third session on Saturday if recovery allows. Optimal training design follows clear structures: 4-6 exercises should be selected per training session, targeting all major muscle groups [s171]. An effective workout must include at least one exercise for the thighs, glutes, chest, shoulders, triceps, back, and biceps [s170]. Specifically, this could mean: squats for legs and glutes, bench press for chest and triceps, pull-ups for back and biceps, and shoulder press for shoulder muscles. Regarding training intensity, for muscle building, 2-5 sets per exercise with 5-15 repetitions are optimal [s170]. The load should feel like an "8 out of 10" on the effort scale [s171]. For beginners, it is advisable to start with a lower intensity (3-4 out of 10) and gradually increase it. Rest periods between sets play an important role and vary depending on the number of repetitions: for 1-3 repetitions, 3-5 minutes of rest are needed, while 8-12 repetitions require 1-2 minutes [s170]. A practical tip: use the rest periods to document your training performance to monitor progress. The principle of progressive overload is fundamental for continuous progress [s172]. This means that the training load must be systematically increased—whether through more weight, additional repetitions, or shorter rest periods. A concrete example: if you can easily perform 12 repetitions of an exercise, increase the weight by 2.5-5% in the next training session. Recovery is an often underestimated aspect of training. Each muscle group requires at least 48 hours of rest [s172], as actual muscle building occurs during the recovery phase [s173]. Practically, this means: do not train the same muscle group on consecutive days and ensure adequate sleep. A successful training program requires regular adjustments and reviews [s174]. Document your training sessions in detail and check your progress every 4-6 weeks. If progress stalls or plateaus, you should incorporate variations [s172]—for example, by changing the order of exercises, introducing new exercises, or adjusting the number of repetitions. In case of unexpected pain or discomfort, it is important to reduce training intensity [s171]. A temporary setback is better than a training-related injury that could lead to a longer forced break.

Glossary

SMART
An acronym from project management that stands for Specific, Measurable, Achievable, Relevant, and Time-bound. This method helps to formulate goals precisely and realistically.

4. 1. 2. Gymnastics

he gymnastics of the horse is a fundamental building block for targeted muscle building and the improvement of overall fitness [s175]. It encompasses various training methods that systematically build upon each other, promoting both the physical and mental development of the horse. An effective gymnastics program begins with foundational work at the walk. This gait is excellent for correcting postural issues and reprogramming the neuromuscular system [s176]. Practically, this means that you should initially work your horse for 15-20 minutes at the walk, paying particular attention to a consistent contact and active engagement of the hind legs. Work at the trot forms the next stage and is particularly effective for improving cardiovascular fitness and muscle tone [s176]. You should ensure that your horse works in a steady rhythm, with trot phases initially not lasting longer than 5-10 minutes. A practical tip is to incorporate hill work: trotting uphill promotes positive stretching of the neck and the gymnastics of the back and hindquarter muscles [s177]. Lateral exercises such as shoulder-in and traverses are important elements for lateral flexibility and muscle development [s178]. Start these exercises at the walk and gradually increase the demands. A proven method is double lungeing, which improves the horse's suppleness and impulsion [s178]. The horse should initially be worked on the long line in both directions before more complex figures are introduced. Working with cavaletti is an extremely effective means of targeted muscle strengthening [s176]. Begin with single poles at the walk and gradually increase the number and height of the cavaletti. A typical progression program might look like this: Week 1-2: 4-6 poles at the walk, Week 3-4: transition to trot over 4 poles, from Week 5: increase the number to 6-8 poles. Monitoring heart rate is an important tool for controlling training intensity [s179]. After intense work sessions, the heart rate should normalize to 60-64 beats per minute within 2-3 minutes. If this does not occur, the training intensity must be adjusted.

For the development of jumping muscles, gymnastic jumping is a sport-specific method that improves both muscle strength and mental and physical agility [s180]. Start with individual small jumps and gradually build combinations. Recovery plays a central role in gymnastics [s181]. Plan sufficient recovery phases after intense training sessions. A balanced training schedule could look like this: Day 1: Dressage work with lateral exercises,

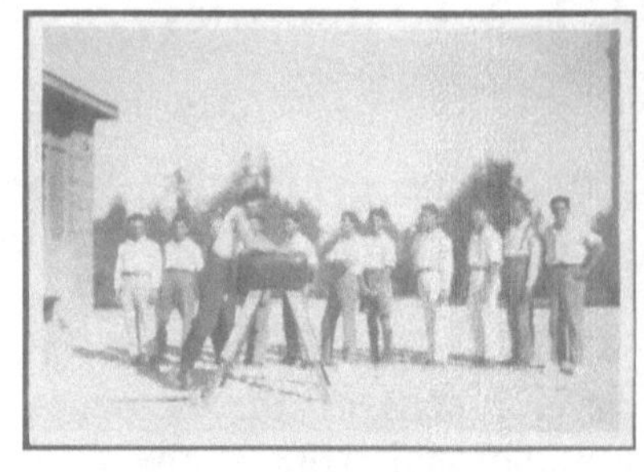

gymnastic jumping [i62]

Day 2: Cavaletti training, Day 3: light movement or rest, Day 4: conditioning work on the hill, Day 5: gymnastic jumping. Regular documentation of training progress is essential [s179]. Record heart rates, recovery times, and qualitative observations regarding movement quality. This allows for an objective assessment of development and aids in adjusting the training program.

Glossary

Cardiovascular

Refers to the heart (cardio) and blood vessels (vascular) and their interplay in the body.

Cavaletti

Special ground poles on adjustable supports used in horse training to improve rhythm, coordination, and movement flow.

Neuromuscular

Describes the interaction between nerves and muscles in movement control.

Traverse

A lateral movement of the horse, where it moves forward-laterally along two tracks, with the body bent in the direction of movement.

4. 1. 3. Strength Building

trength building in horses is a complex physiological process that is regulated at the molecular level through various mechanisms. Muscle hypertrophy, which refers to the enlargement of muscle fibers, primarily occurs through the increase of protein filaments in muscle cells [s182]. Two types of hypertrophy play a significant role: myofibrillar and sarcoplasmic hypertrophy [s182]. A crucial factor for strength building is the protein myostatin, which acts as a natural regulator of muscle growth [s183]. Studies have shown that myostatin expression significantly decreases after targeted training, leading to enhanced muscle fiber enlargement. This is particularly interesting for practical training design, as different genotypes respond differently to training [s183]. Therefore, an individually tailored training program is of great importance. The development of the back muscles shows various temporal phases: hypertrophy of certain back muscles can already be detected in the short-term range. After about 30 days of continuous training, the total cross-sectional area of the back muscles progressively increases on both sides of the body [s184]. A practical approach would be to plan the training in 4-week blocks and document the development through regular measurements of muscle circumferences. For effective strength building, nutrition is fundamentally important. Muscle proteins are built from amino acids, with essential amino acids such as methionine, lysine, and threonine playing a key role [s185]. A practical tip is to specifically feed these nutrients around the time of training. For example, the horse should receive a protein-rich meal about 1-2 hours before training. The topline of the horse deserves special attention, as it is crucial for load-bearing capacity and movement quality [s186]. A weak topline can have various causes, from lack of movement to digestive issues. To address this specifically, a holistic approach is recommended: in addition to training, digestive health and protein supply should also be optimized. A practical example would be the integration of uphill work combined with adjusted protein supplementation. The activation of satellite cells plays an important role in muscle hypertrophy [s183]. This is stimulated by targeted training, where the intensity and frequency of the load must be carefully dosed. A proven training protocol could look as follows: three training sessions per week with progressive increases in intensity, allowing at least one day of rest between intense sessions. Muscle development requires time and patience

[s186]. Depending on the horse's initial condition, progress may become visible at different rates. Regular documentation of development is important, for example through photos from various perspectives or measurements of muscle circumferences. This documentation not only aids in success monitoring but also allows for targeted adjustments to the training program. In addition to protein supply, vitamins and antioxidants also play a significant role, especially during and after intense training sessions [s185]. A balanced nutrition concept should therefore provide these micronutrients in sufficient quantities alongside high-quality proteins. In practice, this means, for example, adding vitamin E and selenium to support muscle recovery.

4. 1. 4. Recovery

ecovery is a complex physiological process that is crucial for successful muscle building and the performance of the horse. It occurs in various phases and can be optimized through targeted measures [s187]. The recovery process after intense training or injuries is divided into three main phases: the inflammatory phase, the regeneration phase, and the remodeling phase [s187]. Particularly important is the adherence to sufficient recovery times—one single day between intense training sessions is demonstrably insufficient to ensure complete tissue healing [s188]. A practical approach is to integrate at least two rest days after intense training sessions. Nutrition plays a key role in the recovery phase. <u>L-Carnitine</u> supplementation has proven particularly effective in shortening recovery time and enabling a quicker return to training [s188]. A specific example of supplementation would be administering L-Carnitine about 30 minutes before training and immediately after exertion. Modern regenerative therapy approaches offer promising possibilities to support healing processes. Three main methods have proven particularly effective [s189]: 1. Platelet-rich plasma (<u>PRP</u>): This therapy improves cell migration and proliferation and optimizes matrix synthesis. In practice, it is often used for tendon injuries. 2. Interleukin-1 receptor antagonist protein: This treatment reduces inflammatory processes and is particularly suitable for degenerative joint diseases. 3. Stem cell therapy: It supports the regeneration of damaged tissue by reducing inflammation and promoting angiogenesis. An innovative method to support tissue regeneration is whole-body vibration [s187]. This therapy improves blood circulation and accelerates the healing process. A practical application example would be a 10-minute vibration therapy session after training, followed by a light massage. For optimal rehabilitation after injuries or intense training phases, a structured program that combines rest and targeted exercises is recommended [s190]. The combination of regular massage and the use of muscle-building supplements can significantly shorten the rehabilitation time. Recent research shows interesting developments in the field of <u>peptide therapy</u> [s191]. Injectable peptides can particularly improve muscle regeneration in older horses by enhancing the immune response and inhibiting pro-fibrotic processes. However, this treatment should only be carried out in consultation with a veterinarian. An often underestimated aspect of recovery is the quality of tissue healing. Poor remodeling can lead to randomly aligned tissue cells, which impairs the structural integrity and elasticity of the tissue [s187]. To avoid this, a gradual and controlled resumption of training is essential. The combination of various regenerative therapies can further improve healing outcomes. For example, the combination of PRP treatment with extracorporeal shock wave therapy shows promising results through the enhanced release of growth factors [s189].

Glossary

L-Carnitine
A naturally occurring substance that helps transport fatty acids into the mitochondria, thereby supporting energy production from fats.

Peptide therapy
A treatment method using short protein chains that can specifically influence certain metabolic processes in the body.

Platelet-rich plasma
A blood component obtained through centrifugation that contains a high concentration of platelets. These are rich in growth factors and can accelerate healing.

Summary - 4. 1. Muscle Building

- The training intensity for optimal muscle development is 2-5 sets with 5-15 repetitions and a subjective load of 8/10.
- For 1-3 repetitions, a rest period of 3-5 minutes is necessary, while 1-2 minutes is sufficient for 8-12 repetitions.
- Each muscle group requires at least 48 hours of recovery for effective muscle growth.
- The heart rate should normalize to 60-64 beats within 2-3 minutes after intense sessions.
- Muscle hypertrophy occurs through myofibrillar and sarcoplasmic mechanisms.
- The protein myostatin acts as a natural regulator of muscle growth.
- After 30 days of continuous training, the total cross-sectional area of the back muscles progressively increases.
- The amino acids methionine, lysine, and threonine play a key role in muscle development.
- The activation of satellite cells is essential for muscle hypertrophy.
- L-carnitine supplementation has been shown to shorten recovery time.
- Platelet-rich plasma (PRP) enhances cell migration and matrix synthesis.
- The combination of PRP with shockwave therapy amplifies the release of growth factors.

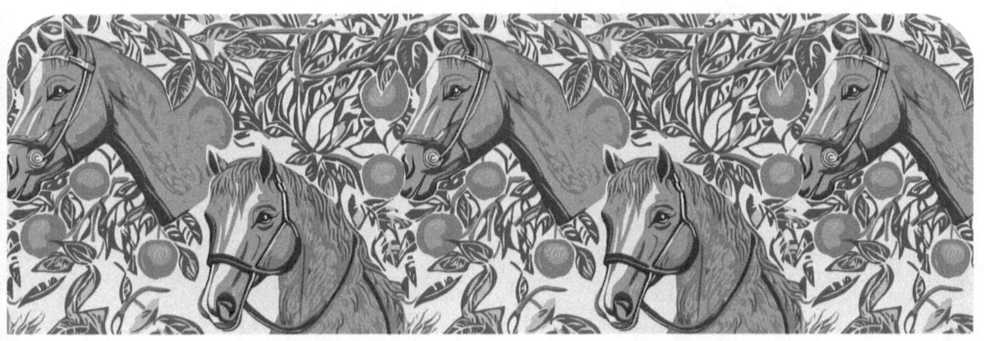

4. 2. Movement Theory

he study of movement in horses raises fascinating questions: How does a horse coordinate its complex movement patterns? What biomechanical principles enable it to switch between different gaits? And how does the sensitive interplay between muscles, the nervous system, and the skeleton develop? Scientific research into equine movement patterns has made significant progress in recent years. From the discovery of genetic factors to the understanding of neurological control processes, knowledge about the movement physiology of horses is steadily increasing. Nevertheless, many aspects, particularly in the area of coordinated fine-tuning and balance regulation, remain to be explored. For horse owners, trainers, and veterinarians, understanding movement science is of fundamental importance. It forms the basis for species-appropriate training, effective therapy, and preventive health care. The following sections illuminate the key aspects of equine movement science and demonstrate how this knowledge can be applied in practice.

„At moderate speeds, horses exhibit a great variation in movement patterns - from the diagonal pattern in the trot to the lateral pattern in the pace."

4. 2. 1. Gaits

he gaits of the horse are complex, rhythmic movement patterns characterized by precise coordination of the limbs and the entire body [s192]. Essentially, a distinction is made between symmetrical and asymmetrical gaits, with the walk, trot, and tölt belonging to the symmetrical category, while the gallop is classified as an asymmetrical gait [s192]. A complete movement cycle consists of various phases: the stance phase, in which the hoof makes contact with the ground, the swing phase, and the suspension phase [s193]. In the stance phase, experts differentiate between an initial deceleration phase and a subsequent propulsion phase, which can be separated at the mid-stance position [s193]. An experienced rider can distinctly feel these phases and should consider them in the training of the horse. Every healthy horse masters the basic gaits of walk (slow) and gallop (fast) [s194]. Interestingly, there is a significant variation in movement patterns at moderate speeds—from the diagonal pattern in the trot to the lateral pattern in the pace [s194]. When assessing gait quality, the temporal coordination of hoof sequence plays a crucial role [s195]. Riders and trainers should pay particular attention to the regularity of the footfall. A special feature is represented by the so-called gaited horses, which are characterized by additional gaits at moderate speeds [s194]. A distinctive characteristic of these special gaits is the "three-foot support"—a moment when three hooves are in contact with the ground simultaneously [s194]. This ability is genetically determined and is controlled by central pattern generators in the spinal cord [s194]. The genetic component of gaits has been further elucidated by the discovery of the DMRT3 mutation [s196]. This mutation plays an important role in the development of various horse breeds with special gaits [s196]. Breeders can now selectively breed for specific gait predispositions through genetic testing [s194]. For practical work with horses, understanding the stride parameters is essential. The stride frequency is measured in steps per second or Hertz [s192]. In training, it should be noted that the accuracy of movement sequences decreases with increasing speed [s195]. This is particularly relevant when working with young or inexperienced horses. Alternative gaits such as pace or various forms of ambling exhibit specific footfall patterns [s196]. In pace, for example, the legs on one side of the body move synchronously, while in trot, the diagonal pairs of legs work together [s196]. These differences should be taken into account in training and conditioning. For the health of the horse, it is important to respect and promote natural movement patterns. Monitoring the temporal stride parameters can help detect irregularities early [s195]. Modern technologies such as <u>inertial measurement units</u> (IMUs) support the precise analysis of movement sequences [s195]. Particular attention should be paid to the development of the basic gaits before training special or artificial gaits. The quality of movement is particularly evident in the regularity and harmony of the stride sequences [s192]. It should be noted that the stance and swing phases should be in a balanced ratio [s193].

Glossary

DMRT3 Mutation
Genetic alteration on chromosome 23, known as 'gait gene', which enables the ability to perform additional gaits such as tölt or pace.

Inertial Measurement Unit
Electronic sensors for measuring acceleration, rotation, and direction of movement. Allow detailed analysis of horse movement without video technology.

Suspension Phase
Phase in the horse's movement cycle during which no hoof is in contact with the ground - also known as the floating phase. Particularly noticeable in trot and gallop.

4. 2. 2. Coordination

oordination in horses is a complex interplay of various systems that goes far beyond mere muscle activity. It is based on the precise interaction of the brain, spinal cord, and musculoskeletal system [s197]. This is particularly evident in the fluid transitions between different gaits, which require a highly precise coordination of all involved systems. The postural control plays a central role in this context. It encompasses various sensory-motor processes responsible for balance in both static and dynamic situations [s198]. For example, a horse must continuously adjust its center of gravity when transitioning from walk to trot, which is only possible through excellent coordination. Riders can support these transitions by initially working within the horse's comfort zone and gradually increasing the demands [s199]. The proprioception, or the perception of one's body position in space, is fundamental to coordination performance. Impairment of this ability can lead to significant coordination disorders and loss of strength [s200]. In practice, this is evident when a horse needs to be rehabilitated after an injury. It is advisable to start with simple coordination exercises on firm, level ground and only gradually increase the complexity. Interestingly, changes in gait serve not only energy efficiency but also stability. Scientific studies have shown that the transition from walk to trot increases robustness against lateral disturbances [s197]. This explains why horses often prefer to trot over walking in uneven terrain. For riders and trainers, this means they should consider this natural tendency when working in the field and allow the horse to choose its gait when it comes to stability and safety. Coordination can be improved through targeted therapeutic interventions [s198]. It is important to stimulate various sensory channels. In practice, exercises with different ground conditions, $1 work, or riding over ground poles have proven effective. These exercises not only promote coordination but also help identify and correct hidden compensation patterns [s199]. From the basic gait "trot," nine different gaits can be developed by varying body inclination and leg loading [s201]. This illustrates the enormous adaptability of the equine musculoskeletal system. For training, this means that a gradual development of coordination skills is possible, always taking into account the individual predisposition and physical condition of the horse. The neurological component of coordination should not be underestimated. Disruptions in signal transmission between the brain and muscles can significantly impair coordination performance [s200]. Regular veterinary check-ups are therefore essential to detect and treat neurological problems early. For practical work with horses, this means that a systematic development of coordination skills is essential. The approach should follow the principle of "from easy to difficult" and "from simple to complex." It is particularly important to give the horse sufficient time to develop its coordination skills and to avoid overexertion.

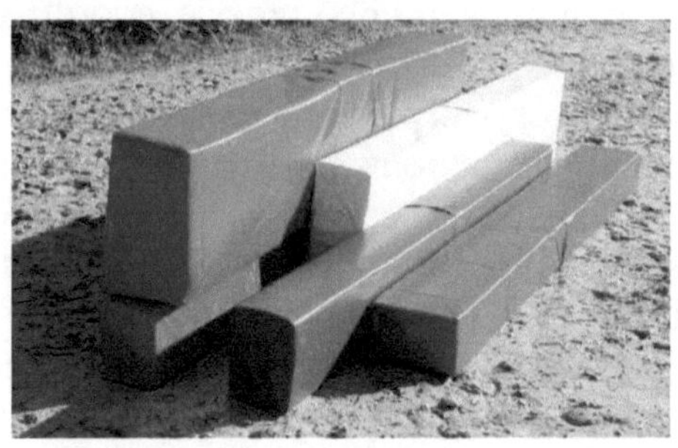

Cavaletti [i63]

Glossary

Postural

Refers to body posture and its control. A system of reflexes and muscle activities that regulates the upright position and balance of the body.

4. 2. 3. Balance

he balance of a horse is fundamental to its health, performance, and harmonious interaction with the rider. A balanced horse can move efficiently and is less prone to injuries [s202]. The development and maintenance of balance is a complex process that encompasses various aspects of <u>biomechanics</u> and movement control. An important principle is that true strength can only be built on the foundation of stability. When a horse tries to find its balance or adopts a crooked posture, it cannot develop the kind of strength that leads to improved performance [s202]. In practical work, this means that stability must be addressed first before focusing on strength exercises. This can be achieved through targeted exercises for foot placement and control of the vertebral joints. The biomechanics of the horse is based on four dimensions of movement that should be considered in a modern, horse-friendly training system [s203]. It is important for the rider to understand how these dimensions interact. A practical approach is to start with simple weight-shifting exercises and gradually develop them into more complex movements. The alignment of the rider plays a crucial role in the horse's balance. The rider's shoulders should be relaxed and aligned directly over the pelvis [s204]. A stable and straight horse's back facilitates the rider's perception of their own position. In practice, it is advisable to regularly check one's own seating position and improve it through targeted exercises if necessary. Interesting insights come from hippotherapy: The rhythmic movement impulses originating from the horse's back stimulate the <u>postural reflex mechanisms</u> [s205]. This insight can also be applied to the training of healthy horses. Through targeted training, the synchronization between the movements of the horse and the rider can be improved [s206], leading to better functional mobility. Working on the suppleness of the horse is an essential first step towards improving straightness [s204]. Practical exercises can initially be performed while standing before being transferred to movement. Special attention should be paid to the even loading of both sides of the body, as asymmetries can lead to reduced core strength. An important aspect of balance is the horse's body awareness. To achieve stability, the horse needs improved awareness and control over its foot placement as well as the ability to maintain the alignment of its vertebral joints during movement [s202]. This can be promoted through specific groundwork exercises where the horse learns to place its feet purposefully and control its body consciously. The development of balance should occur systematically and without time pressure. Scientific studies show that stability improves with increased practice, which is reflected in a reduction of deviations in the center of pressure [s205]. For trainers and riders, this means they should give their horses sufficient time to develop and solidify new movement patterns.

Glossary

Biomechanics
The science that deals with the mechanical laws in living organisms. In horses, it examines the forces and movements acting on bones, joints, and muscles.

Postural Reflex Mechanisms
Automatic body reactions that serve to maintain posture and balance. These reflexes are controlled by sensory organs in the inner ear, muscles, and joints.

Summary - 4. 2. Movement Theory

- The DMRT3 mutation significantly determines the ability for specific gaits such as tölt or pace. Gaited horses are characterized by a distinctive 'three-foot support' at moderate speeds. The accuracy of movement patterns systematically decreases with increasing speed. The transition from walk to trot demonstrably increases robustness against lateral disturbances. From the basic gait 'trot,' nine different gaits can be developed by varying body inclination. Postural control encompasses sensory-motor processes for static and dynamic balance. Impairment of proprioception leads to measurable loss of strength and coordination disorders. The rhythmic movement impulses of the horse's back directly stimulate postural reflex mechanisms. Asymmetries in movement result in a measurable reduction in core strength. Stability improves with increased practice, measurable by reduced deviations of the center of pressure. True strength development is only possible on the basis of stable balance, not in compensatory postures.

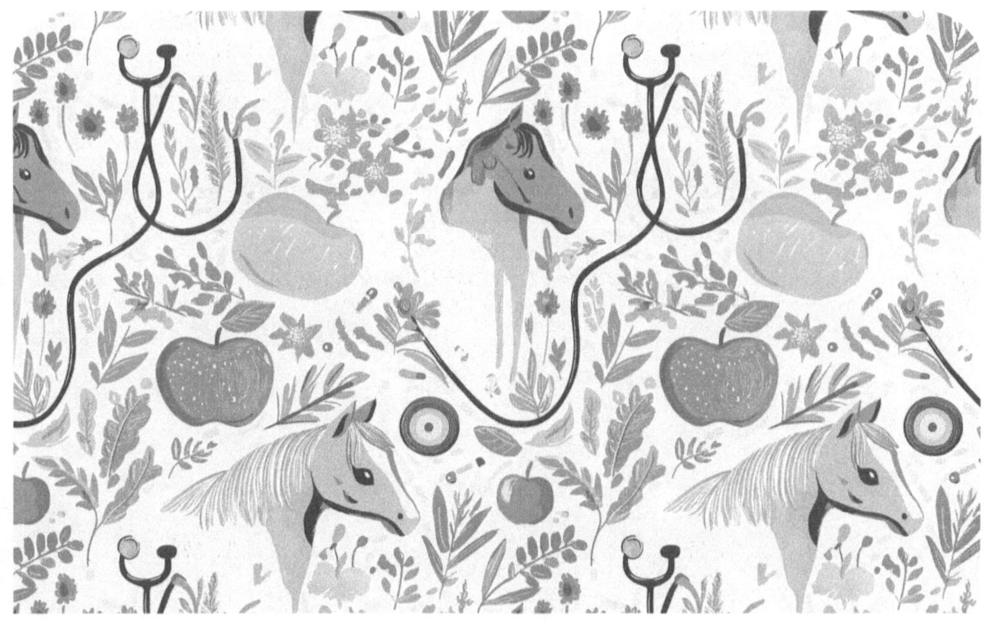

4. 3. Performance Optimization

he optimization of athletic performance in horses raises complex questions: How can training be designed to be both effective and health-preserving? Which physiological parameters must be considered to avoid overexertion? And how can systematic training planning contribute to injury prevention? Recent scientific research has shown that performance optimization in horses requires a finely tuned interplay of load management, structured training planning, and preventive measures. Both measurable parameters such as heart rate and lactate levels, as well as the individual constitution of the horse, play a crucial role. The challenge lies in finding the right balance between training stimuli and recovery—a task that necessitates a solid understanding of training physiology fundamentals. The following sections illustrate how modern insights from sports physiology can be integrated into practical training work.

„The 80/20 rule states that approximately 80% of training should occur in the low-intensity range to ensure sustainable performance development."

4. 3. 1. Load Management

Professional load management is a central component for the sustainable performance development and health maintenance of sport horses. It is based on the systematic monitoring and adjustment of training stimuli, taking into account both physiological and biomechanical parameters [s207]. A fundamental principle of load management is the 80/20 rule, which states that approximately 80% of training should occur in the low-intensity range [s208]. This is particularly important for the long-term development of young horses, where early overexertion must be avoided. A practical example would be the design of a typical training week: out of five training days, four should be in the moderate intensity range, while only one day is designated for high-intensity training. Heart rate monitoring plays a central role in load management. Studies have shown that horses with lower heart rates during the warm-up phase and higher maximum heart rates during intense exertion phases perform better [s209]. For trainers, this means that they should keep an eye on their horses' heart rates during warm-up—ideally, this should be at 40-50% of the maximum heart rate during the warm-up phase. Heart rate variability (<u>HRV</u>) has established itself as an important indicator for training control [s210]. Trainers should regularly measure their horses' HRV values in the morning at rest. A significant drop in HRV may indicate overexertion and should lead to an immediate reduction in training intensity. Special attention is required for rehabilitation after injuries. The use of dynamic support systems has proven effective, allowing for precise control of the load [s211]. These systems enable a gradual increase in load, for example, through controlled restriction of fetlock joint extension during various movement phases. Monitoring blood lactate levels has proven to be a particularly meaningful parameter for assessing training adaptation [s212]. Trainers should conduct regular lactate measurements during standardized exertion tests to determine the individual anaerobic threshold of their horses and adjust training accordingly. A common mistake in training practice is underestimating signs of overtraining. Studies have shown that the fitness of sport horses can decrease during intense training phases [s213]. Therefore, trainers should establish a systematic monitoring process that considers not only performance parameters but also behavioral changes and recovery times. For practical implementation, it is advisable to maintain a detailed training diary, in which not only objective measurements but also subjective observations are recorded [s207]. This allows for the recognition of long-term trends and the adjustment of training accordingly. A proven scheme is the weekly evaluation of the collected data followed by training adjustments for the upcoming week. The individual adaptability of horses must be particularly considered. Interestingly, studies show that horses with initially poorer performance parameters often achieve the greatest training progress [s212]. This underscores the importance of a patient and systematic approach to performance development. For optimal load management, it is essential to capture both external (e.g., training volume, intensity) and internal load parameters (e.g., heart rate, lactate levels) and relate them to each other [s207]. This allows for precise tuning of training load to the individual fitness level of the horse and helps find the optimal balance between load and recovery.

Glossary

Heart Rate Variability
The time interval between individual heartbeats, which provides insight into the adaptability of the heart and the interplay between the sympathetic and parasympathetic nervous systems.

Lactate
A metabolic byproduct that occurs during intense muscle work without sufficient oxygen supply and can lead to muscle acidosis.

4. 3. 2. Training Planning

A systematic training plan is fundamental for the successful performance development of sport horses. The planning follows the principle of periodization, which structures various training cycles and phases in a coherent manner [s214]. The foundation is the basic training, characterized by longer, moderate training sessions. In this phase, the focus is on developing aerobic capacity and building basic endurance [s215]. A typical training block might consist of three 45-minute sessions per week, during which the horse is primarily exercised at a trot and a light gallop. Following the foundational phase, a systematic increase occurs through the integration of specific training stimuli. Here, interval training and targeted speed sessions are increasingly employed [s216]. A proven interval training regimen might look as follows: after a 15-minute warm-up, 4-6 intervals of 2-3 minutes at increased intensity are followed by 3-4 minutes of active recovery at a walk. Particular importance is given to the concept of "Peaking", which refers to the targeted management of form leading up to a competition peak [s217]. About two weeks before important competitions, a Tapering phase is initiated, during which the training volume is reduced by 40-90%, while the intensity of the remaining sessions remains high. This strategy can enhance competition performance by 3-6%. The Block Periodization has proven to be an effective concept, where specific training goals are addressed in concentrated blocks [s214]. A typical 4-week block might initially focus on endurance, followed by a week of intensive strength training, a week of speed training, and a recovery week.

For practical implementation, a balanced relationship between load and recovery is essential [s216]. Trainers should adhere to the following basic rules:
- At least one complete rest day per week
- Variation between intensive and restorative training sessions
- Regular monitoring of recovery ability through observation of behavioral patterns and vital parameters

The integration of mental training into the training plan is gaining increasing importance [s216]. For instance, quiet rides in nature or targeted relaxation exercises during recovery phases can be incorporated. An often underestimated aspect is the balance between strength and endurance training [s215]. This can be practically implemented through the integration of hill work or controlled uphill gallops for strength development, while longer trot phases on flat ground serve endurance development.

The training plan must also consider the individual needs and adaptability of the horse [s214]. Trainers should establish a detailed monitoring system that includes the following aspects:
- Daily documentation of training content and volume
- Regular recording of performance parameters
- Logging of recovery times and behavioral anomalies

Nutrition plays an important supportive role in training planning [s216]. The nutrition plan should be adjusted to the respective training phase, with energy requirements needing to be increased during intensive phases. For long-term development, it is important to integrate regular testing sessions into the plan to assess training success and make adjustments as necessary. These tests should be conducted under standardized conditions to obtain comparable results.

Glossary

Block Periodization
A modern training concept where different training goals are trained in concentrated, consecutive time periods, rather than developing multiple skills in parallel.

Peaking
A training method from competitive sports, where the performance peak is precisely reached at the desired time through targeted management of training load.

Tapering
A training technique in which the training load is systematically reduced before a competition to alleviate fatigue and achieve optimal performance.

4. 3. 3. Injury Prevention

njury prevention is a complex and important topic in equestrian sports, as approximately 16% of sport horses are affected by significant soft tissue injuries each year, leading to training interruptions [s218]. A systematic prevention approach is therefore essential for the long-term health of the horses. The $1 plays a central role in injury prevention. Trainers must thoroughly understand the specific demands of their discipline, as most training-related injuries are avoidable with correct biomechanical understanding [s219]. A practical example: In dressage horses, particular attention should be paid to the even distribution of weight on both sides of the body. This can be achieved through regular changes of rein and balanced work sessions on both reins. Repeated overload has been identified as a primary cause of soft tissue injuries [s218]. This often arises from a combination of fatigue, existing lameness, and unfavorable conformation. To counteract this, the integration of cross-training into the training plan is recommended [s220]. An effective cross-training program could consist of a combination of dressage work, controlled terrain sessions, and gymnastic work on the lunge. The ground conditions play a crucial role in injury prevention [s221]. Trainers should systematically acclimatize their horses to different surfaces [s220]. A practical approach would be to structure the training as follows: warming up on firm, level ground, main working phase on the respective discipline-specific surface, and relaxation phase back on firm ground. Modern technologies offer innovative possibilities for injury prevention. In particular, shock wave therapy, infrared thermography, and electrotherapies have proven effective in preventing muscle contractures [s222]. However, these methods should always be used in consultation with the attending veterinarian.

An often underestimated aspect is the importance of the horse's core strength [s220]. Targeted core stabilization training can be achieved through specific exercises. Practical exercises for this include:
- Pole work at walk and trot
- Cavaletti training at various distances
- Work on a slope
- Backing up in a straight line

The housing conditions significantly influence the risk of injury. Studies show that pure stable confinement increases the risk of soft tissue injuries [s218]. A preventive measure is to ensure sufficient movement outside of training, ideally through regular turnout or paddock stays.

A comprehensive prevention program must also include regular monitoring and care of hooves, teeth, and equipment [s219]. A practical monitoring plan could look as follows:
- Daily hoof checks before and after training
- Monthly equipment checks for wear
- Biannual dental check by the veterinarian
- Regular saddle adjustments

The development of educational modules for trainers, owners, and veterinarians is an important component of injury prevention [s221]. These should particularly convey the recognition of early warning signs and the importance of preventive measures. An adequate warm-up and cool-down phase is fundamental for injury prevention [s219]. A structured warm-up program should last at least 15-20 minutes and gradually increase in intensity. The cool-down phase should be similarly long and conclude with relaxed, stretching elements.

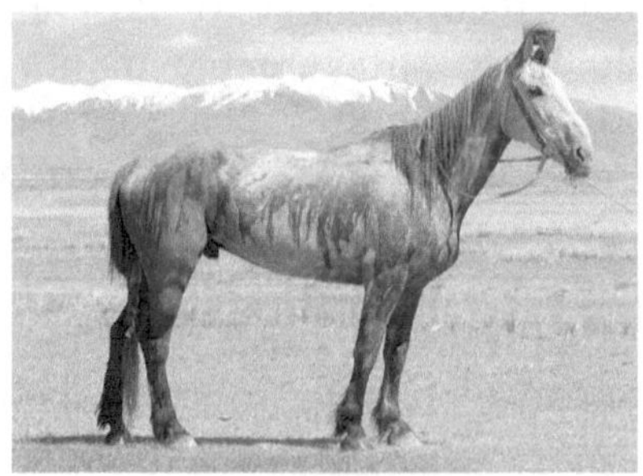

Conformation [i64]

Summary - 4.3. Performance Optimization

- The 80/20 rule states that 80% of training should occur in the low-intensity range.
- Lower heart rates during the warm-up phase correlate with better performance.
- A significant drop in heart rate variability indicates overtraining.
- Dynamic support systems enable precise load control in rehabilitation.
- Horses with initially poorer performance parameters often show the greatest training progress.
- The tapering phase reduces training volume by 40-90% two weeks before competitions.
- Block periodization focuses specific training goals in 4-week blocks.
- 16% of sport horses suffer significant soft tissue injuries annually.
- Cross-training reduces the risk of injury by varying the forms of load.
- Shockwave therapy and infrared thermography have proven effective in preventing muscle contractures.
- Pure stable housing significantly increases the risk of soft tissue injuries.
- The combination of fatigue, existing lameness, and unfavorable conformation is the main cause of soft tissue injuries.

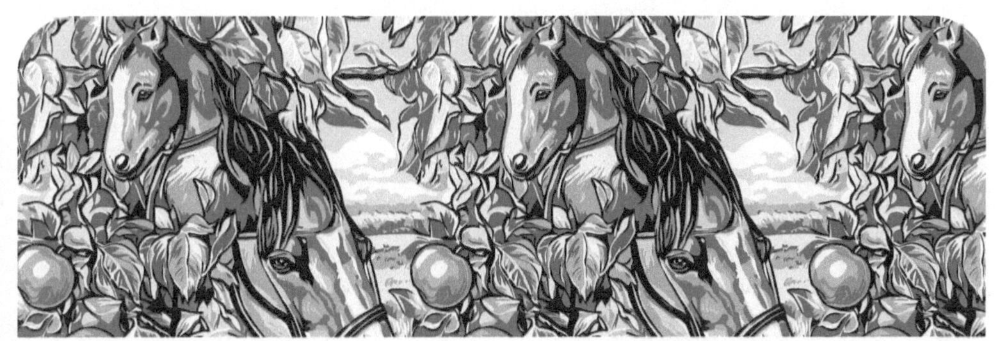

- Muscle hypertrophy occurs through an increase in protein filaments, distinguishing between myofibrillar and sarcoplasmic hypertrophy. The protein myostatin acts as a natural regulator of muscle growth, and its expression significantly decreases after training. The back muscles show a progressive increase in total cross-sectional area after just 30 days of continuous training. The activation of satellite cells plays an important role in muscle hypertrophy and is stimulated by targeted training. Heart rate variability (HRV) has established itself as an important indicator for training control. Block periodization allows for concentrated work on specific training goals within defined time blocks. Approximately 16% of sport horses are affected by significant soft tissue injuries annually. The DMRT3 mutation plays a crucial role in the development of various horse breeds with specific gaits. Postural control encompasses sensory-motor processes for balance in static and dynamic situations. Proprioception is fundamental for coordinated performance, and its impairment leads to coordination disorders. The transition from walk to trot increases robustness against lateral disturbances. Integrating cross-training into the training plan reduces the risk of injury from unilateral loads. Modern technologies such as shockwave therapy and infrared thermography have proven effective in injury prevention. The tapering phase before competitions, with a 40-90% reduction in training volume, can enhance performance by 3-6%.

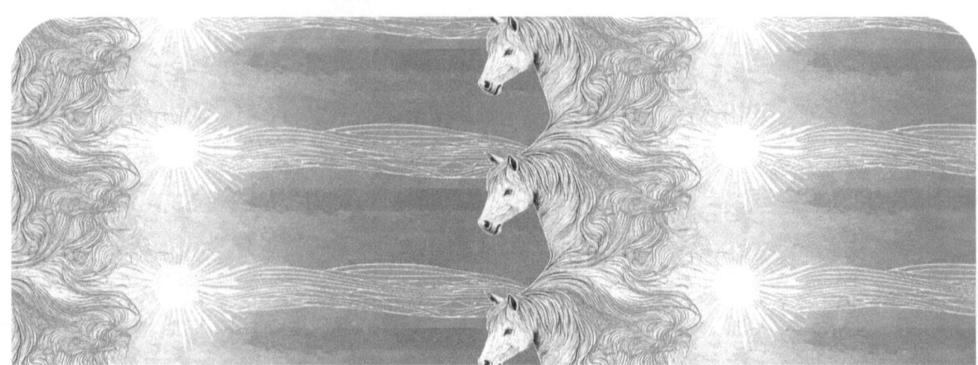

Free Additional Offers Planned

We are pleased to offer you free supplementary materials for this book in the future:

- An exclusive bonus chapter with additional content
- A compact summary of the entire book in PDF format

These materials are expected to be released in January 2025.
Feel free to visit our website today. Once our newsletter service launches (expected January 2025), you can register there for updates and won't miss any news about the free additional offers.

SaageBooks.com/horse_health-bonus-NSXJPU

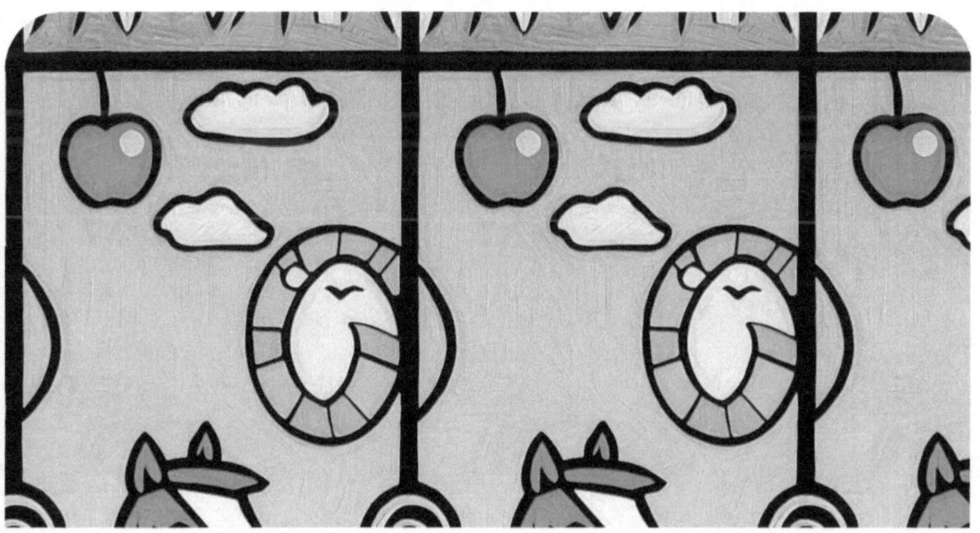

Dear readers,

I am deeply honored that you have taken the time to read my book from beginning to end. As an author, my greatest wish is to provide you with valuable insights and practical guidance. Your trust in my work means a lot to me. I hope the reading was enriching for you. If you have any questions or suggestions, please feel free to contact me through our website.

If you enjoyed this book, I would greatly appreciate an honest review. Your opinion matters to me and helps other readers make their decision. You can easily leave your honest rating on the sales platform where you purchased the book.
Thank you for your support!

Artemis Saage

Saage Media GmbH

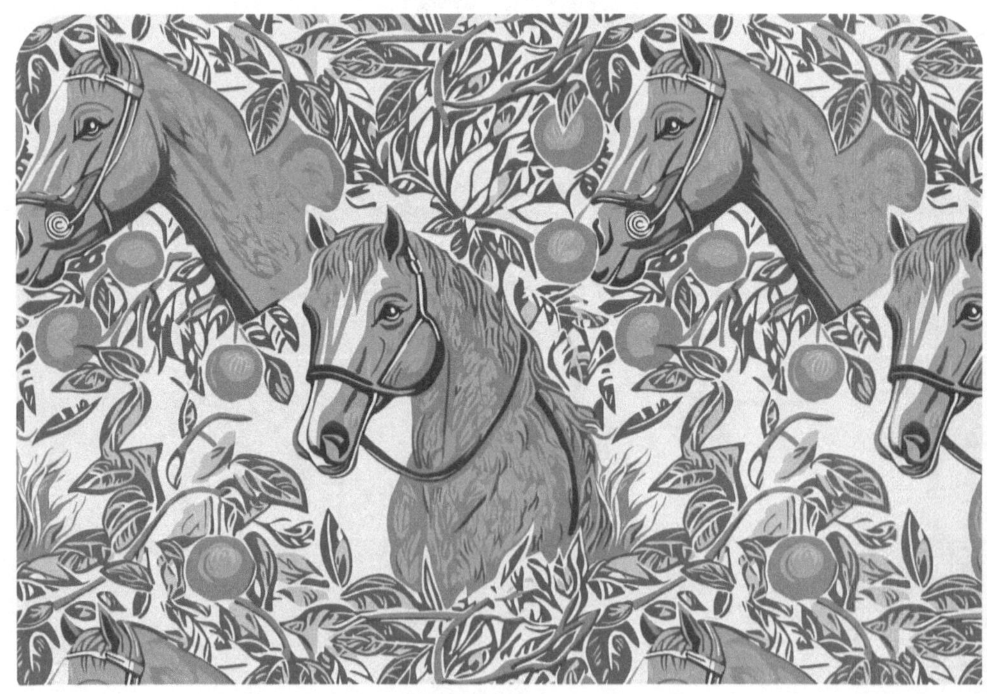

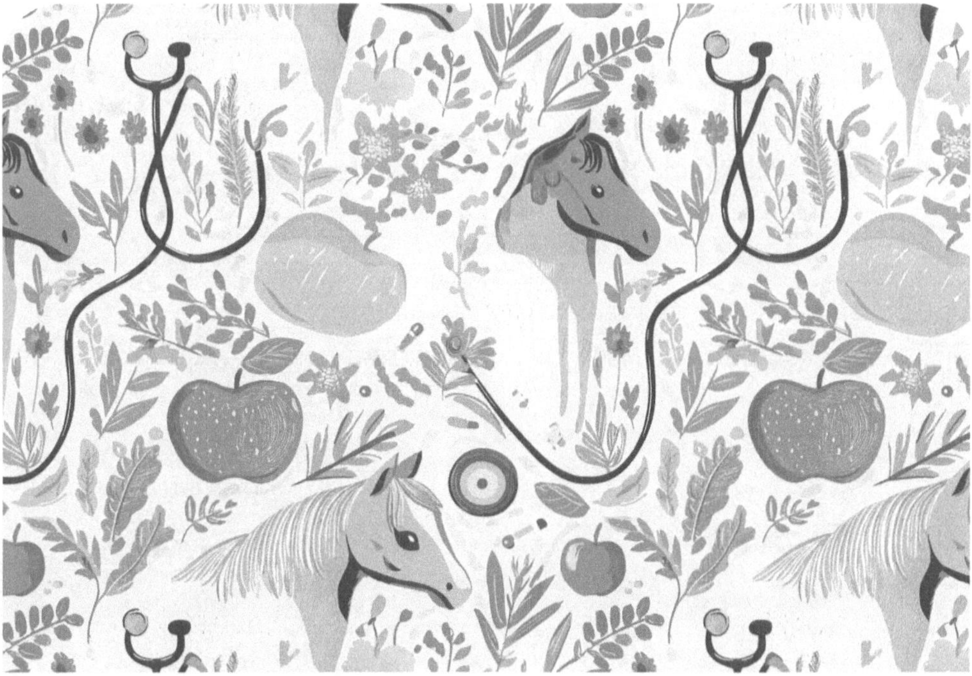

Sources

My sincere thanks go to all authors of the cited scientific and non-scientific sources, the operators of the referenced websites, and the creators of the images, graphics, and studies used, whose valuable work has significantly contributed to the creation of this book.
For more information, I recommend visiting the linked source websites.

All sources were last accessed on: 2024-12-03

[s1] - https://www.nature.com/articles/s41598-024-75960-7
Author: Jindi Wu, Heya Na, Fan Bai, Siyu Li, Hao Gao, Rina Sha — **Title:** Preparation and tissue structure analysis of horse bone collagen peptide
Release Date: 28 October 2024 — **Website:** Nature
Publisher: Scientific Reports

[s2] - https://www.nature.com/articles/s41598-018-29655-5
Author: J. Oinas, A. P. Ronkainen, L. Rieppo, M. A. J. Finnilä, J. T. Iivarinen, P. R. van Weeren, H. J. Helminen, P. A. J. Brama, R. K. Korhonen, S. Saarakkala — **Title:** Composition, structure and tensile biomechanical properties of equine articular cartilage during growth and maturation
by: Nature Research — **Release Date:** 27 July 2018
Website: Nature — **Publisher:** Scientific Reports

[s3] - https://avmajournals.avma.org/downloadpdf/view/journals/ajvr/52/1/ajvr.1991.52.01.133.pdf
Author: David A. Wilson, DVM, MS; Gordon J. Baker, BVSc, PhD; Gerald J. Pijanowski, DVM, PhD; Michael J. Boero, DVM, MS; Robert R. Badertscher II, DVM, PhD — **Title:** Composition and morphologic features of the interosseous muscle in Standardbreds and Thoroughbreds
Release Date: January 1991 — **Website:** AVMA Journals
Publisher: American Veterinary Medical Association

[s4] - https://optionsforanimals.com/wp-content/uploads/2019/02/Ex_and_Tx_of_Eq_Back_Pain.pdf
Author: Kevin K. Haussler, DVM, DC, PhD — **Title:** Review of the Examination and Treatment of Back and Pelvic Disorders
by: Gail Holmes Equine Orthopaedic Research Center, Colorado State University — **Website:** optionsforanimals.com
Publisher: American Association of Equine Practitioners

[s5] - https://www.mdpi.com/2076-2615/11/1/234
Author: Gravrok, J., et al. — **Title:** Beyond the Benefits of Assistance Dogs: Exploring Challenges Experienced by First-Time Handlers
by: MDPI — **Release Date:** 2019
Website: MDPI — **Publisher:** MDPI

[s6] - https://www.nature.com/articles/s41598-020-65339-9
Author: Ryotaro Nagakura, Masahito Yamamoto, Juhee Jeong, Nobuyuki Hinata, Yukio Katori, Wei-Jen Chang, Shinichi Abe — **Title:** Switching of Sox9 expression during musculoskeletal system development
by: Nature Publishing Group — **Release Date:** 2020-05-21
Website: Nature — **Publisher:** Scientific Reports

[s7] - https://www.ivis.org/sites/default/files/library/aaep/1997/Haussler.pdf
Author: Kevin K. Haussler, DVM, DC, PhD — **Title:** Application of Chiropractic Principles and Techniques to Equine Practice
Release Date: 1997 — **Website:** IVIS
Publisher: AAEP

[s8] - https://www.epauk.org/about-equine-podiatry/articles/hoof-anatomy-a-beginners-guide/
Title: Hoof Anatomy – A Beginner's Guide — **by:** Equine Podiatry Association
Website: Equine Podiatry Association

[s9] - https://extension.missouri.edu/sites/default/files/legacy_media/wysiwyg/Extensiondata/Pub/pdf/agguides/ansci/g02740.pdf
Author: Robert C. McClure, Gerald R. Kirk, Phillip D. Garrett — **Title:** Functional Anatomy of the Horse Foot
by: University of Missouri — **Release Date:** 10/99
Website: MU Extension — **Publisher:** University of Missouri

[s10] - https://equine-jogging-shoes.com/advice-guidance/rubber-sole/
Title: Unique Rubber Sole Benefits — **by:** All Natural Horse Care
Release Date: 2023 — **Website:** Equine Jogging Shoes

[s11] - https://digitalcommons.otterbein.edu/stu_honor/56/
Author: Sharlee Lowe — **Title:** The Effect of Whole Body Vibration on Equine Hoof Growth
Release Date: 2017 — **Website:** Digital Commons @ Otterbein

[s12] - https://pubmed.ncbi.nlm.nih.gov/7988538/
Author: P Dyhre-Poulsen, H H Smedegaard, J Roed, E Korsgaard — **Title:** Equine hoof function investigated by pressure transducers inside the hoof and accelerometers mounted on the first phalanx
Release Date: 1994-09 — **Website:** PubMed
Publisher: Equine Veterinary Journal

[s13] - https://www.extension.purdue.edu/extmedia/id/id-321-w.pdf
Author: Kate Hepworth, Dr. Michael Neary, Dr. Simon Kenyon
Title: Hoof Anatomy, Care and Management in Livestock
by: Purdue University Cooperative Extension Service
Release Date: 10/04
Website: Purdue University Extension
Publisher: Purdue University Cooperative Extension Service

[s14] - https://www.equestriansurfaces.co.uk/news/horse-hoof-anatomy-your-complete-guide/
Title: Horse Hoof Anatomy: Your Complete Guide
by: Equestrian Surfaces
Release Date: 06.03.2023
Website: Equestrian Surfaces

[s15] - https://nebraskaequine.com/about-us/our-services/chiropractic-and-acupuncture.html
Title: Chiropractic and Acupuncture
by: Nebraska Equine Veterinary Clinic
Website: Nebraska Equine Veterinary Clinic

[s16] - https://vet.arioneo.com/en/blog/horse-back-anatomy-and-biomechanics/
Title: Horse back: anatomy and biomechanics
by: Arioneo
Release Date: 2022-11-18
Website: Arioneo

[s17] - https://www.nature.com/articles/s41598-021-92272-2
Author: A. Byström, A. M. Hardeman, F. M. Serra Braganca, L. Roepstorff, J. H. Swagemakers, P. R. van Weeren, A. Egenvall
Title: Differences in equine spinal kinematics between straight line and circle in trot
by: Nature Publishing Group
Release Date: 2021-06-18
Website: Nature
Publisher: Scientific Reports

[s18] - https://emedicine.medscape.com/article/1899031-overview
Author: Stephen Kishner, MD, MHA; Chief Editor: Thomas R Gest, PhD
Title: Lumbar Spine Anatomy: Overview, Gross Anatomy, Natural Variants
by: Medscape
Release Date: Nov 09, 2017
Website: Medscape

[s19] - https://pubmed.ncbi.nlm.nih.gov/10218240/
Author: J M Denoix
Title: Spinal biomechanics and functional anatomy
by: National Institute of Agronomic Research
Release Date: 1999-04
Website: PubMed
Publisher: Vet Clin North Am Equine Pract

[s20] - https://veteriankey.com/the-respiratory-system-anatomy-physiology-and-adaptations-to-exercise-and-training/
Author: PIERRE LEKEUX, TATIANA ART, DAVID R. HODGSON
Title: The respiratory system: Anatomy, physiology, and adaptations to exercise and training
by: Veterinary Key
Website: Veterinary Key

[s21] - https://vet.ucalgary.ca/community/learning-animal-health/anatomy/equine
Title: Equine Anatomy
by: University of Calgary
Website: University of Calgary Veterinary Medicine

[s22] - https://vethospital.tamu.edu/large-animal/equine-soft-tissue-surgery/respiratory-tract/
Title: Respiratory Tract
by: Texas A&M University
Website: Texas A&M Veterinary Hospital

[s23] - https://www.westvets.com.au/wp-content/uploads/2017/06/respiratory-conditions.pdf
Author: Sarah Van Dyck
Title: Respiratory Conditions Part One
by: WestVETS Animal Hospital & Reproduction Centre
Release Date: March 2016
Website: Horses and People Magazine

[s24] - https://en.audevard.com/blog/the-horse-s-respiratory-system
Title: The horse's respiratory system
by: Audevard Laboratories
Website: Audevard

[s25] - https://extension.umd.edu/resource/teaching-basic-equine-nutrition-part-ii-equine-digestive-anatomy-and-physiology
Author: Amy Burk
Title: Teaching Basic Equine Nutrition Part II: Equine Digestive Anatomy and Physiology
by: University of Maryland Extension
Release Date: September 7, 2021
Website: University of Maryland Extension

[s26] - https://www.ivis.org/sites/default/files/library/aaep/2001/91010100053.pdf
Author: James N. Moore, DVM, PhD; Thel Melton, BA; William C. Carter, MS, CMI; Allison L. Wright, MS, CMI; Malcolm L. Smith, PhD
Title: A New Look at Equine Gastrointestinal Anatomy, Function, and Selected Intestinal Displacements
Release Date: 2001
Website: IVIS
Publisher: AAEP

[s27] - https://extension.umaine.edu/publications/1005e/
Title: Bulletin #1005, Equine Facts: Basic Horse Nutrition
by: University of Maine
Website: University of Maine Cooperative Extension

[s28] - https://pubmed.ncbi.nlm.nih.gov/8800413/
Author: J E Reynolds 3rd, S A Rommel
Title: Structure and function of the gastrointestinal tract of the Florida manatee, Trichechus manatus latirostris
by: Eckerd College
Release Date: 1996-07
Website: PubMed
Publisher: Anatomical Record

[s29] - https://animalmicrobiome.biomedcentral.com/articles/10.1186/s42523-022-00224-6
Author: Georgia Wunderlich, Michelle Bull, Tom Ross, Michael Rose, Belinda Chapman
Title: Understanding the microbial fibre degrading communities & processes in the equine gut
by: BMC (BioMed Central)
Release Date: 2023-01-12
Website: Animal Microbiome
Publisher: BMC (BioMed Central)

[s30] - https://bmcmicrobiol.biomedcentral.com/articles/10.1186/s12866-023-03001-w
Author: Yiping Zhao, Xiujuan Ren, Haiqing Wu, He Hu, Chao Cheng, Ming Du, Yao Huang, Xiaoqing Zhao, Liwei Wang, Liuxi Yi, Jinshan Tao, Yajing Li, Yanan Lin, Shaofeng Su, Manglai Dugarjaviin
Title: Diversity and functional prediction of fungal communities in different segments of mongolian horse gastrointestinal tracts
by: BMC
Release Date: 2023-09-09
Website: BMC Microbiology
Publisher: BMC

[s31] - https://vet.ucalgary.ca/community/learning-animal-health/anatomy/equine
Title: Equine Anatomy
by: University of Calgary
Website: University of Calgary Veterinary Medicine

[s32] - https://pubmed.ncbi.nlm.nih.gov/3877552/
Author: D L Evans
Title: Cardiovascular adaptations to exercise and training
Release Date: 1985-12
Website: PubMed
Publisher: Vet Clin North Am Equine Pract

[s33] - https://pubmed.ncbi.nlm.nih.gov/15134294/
Author: Claus D Buergelt
Title: Equine cardiovascular pathology: an overview
by: University of Florida
Release Date: 2003-12
Website: PubMed
Publisher: Animal Health Research Reviews

[s34] - https://www.mdpi.com/2227-7390/9/20/2580
Title: Computer Simulations of Dynamic Response of Ferrofluids on an Alternating Magnetic Field with High Amplitude
by: MDPI
Website: MDPI
Publisher: MDPI

[s35] - https://www.vetspecialists.com/specialties/cardiology
Title: Cardiology
by: VetSpecialists
Website: VetSpecialists

[s36] - https://pubmed.ncbi.nlm.nih.gov/15134294/
Author: Claus D Buergelt
Title: Equine cardiovascular pathology: an overview
Release Date: 2003-12
Website: PubMed
Publisher: Anim Health Res Rev

[s37] - https://doi.org/10.1186/s12987-020-00230-3
Author: Hossam Kadry, Behnam Noorani, Luca Cucullo
Title: A blood–brain barrier overview on structure, function, impairment, and biomarkers of integrity
Release Date: 2020-11-18
Website: Fluids and Barriers of the CNS
Publisher: BMC

[s38] - https://vanat.ahc.umn.edu/
Author: T.F. Fletcher
Title: Carnivore Anatomy Courseware
by: University of Minnesota College of Veterinary Medicine
Release Date: January 2021
Website: Minnesota Veterinary Anatomy Courseware Web Site

[s39] - https://vetmed.tennessee.edu/vmc/equinehospital/equineacupuncture/
Title: Acupuncture and Chiropractic
by: University of Tennessee Institute of Agriculture
Website: University of Tennessee College of Veterinary Medicine

[s40] - https://equine.ca.uky.edu/news-story/understanding-differences-between-ems-and-ppid
Title: Understanding the Differences between EMS and PPID
by: University of Kentucky
Release Date: June, 2013
Website: University of Kentucky Ag Equine Programs

[s41] - https://cvm.msu.edu/vdl/client-education/guides-for-pet-owners/equine-endocrinology-pituitary-pars-intermedia-dysfunction-ppid
Title: Equine Endocrinology: Pituitary Pars Intermedia Dysfunction (PPID)
by: Michigan State University College of Veterinary Medicine
Website: Veterinary Diagnostic Laboratory

[s42] - https://actavetscand.biomedcentral.com/articles/10.1186/s13028-019-0480-2
Author: Caterina Squillacioti, Alessandra Pelagalli, Giovanna Liguori, Nicola Mirabella
Title: Urocortins in the mammalian endocrine system
by: BMC
Release Date: 2019-10-04
Website: Acta Veterinaria Scandinavica
Publisher: BMC

[s43] - https://avmajournals.avma.org/downloadpdf/view/journals/javma/261/2/javma.22.11.0485.pdf
Author: Jane M. Manfredi, DVM, PhD; Sarah Jacob, DVM, PhD; Elaine Norton, DVM, PhD
Title: Endocrine Disorders: a One-Health Issue
by: Michigan State University; University of Arizona
Release Date: February 2023
Website: avmajournals.avma.org
Publisher: American Veterinary Medical Association

[s44] - https://catalog.uconn.edu/undergraduate/courses/ansc/
Title: Undergraduate Catalog
by: University of Connecticut
Release Date: 2024-2025
Website: University of Connecticut Catalog

[s45] - https://nutritionandmetabolism.biomedcentral.com/articles/10.1186/1743-7075-11-10
Author: Shuai Zhang, Matthew W Hulver, Ryan P McMillan, Mark A Cline, Elizabeth R Gilbert
Title: The pivotal role of pyruvate dehydrogenase kinases in metabolic flexibility
Release Date: 12 February 2014
Website: Nutrition & Metabolism
Publisher: BMC

[s46] - https://pubmed.ncbi.nlm.nih.gov/35968025/
Author: Xiaohui Wen, Shengjun Luo, Dianhong Lv, Chunling Jia, Xiurong Zhou, Qi Zhai, Li Xi, Caijuan Yang
Title: Variations in the fecal microbiota and their functions of Thoroughbred, Mongolian, and Hybrid horses
by: Guangdong Academy of Agricultural Sciences
Release Date: 2022-07-28
Website: PubMed
Publisher: Frontiers in Veterinary Science

[s47] - https://pubmed.ncbi.nlm.nih.gov/35705806/
Author: Veronica L Li, Yang He, Kévin Contrepois, Hailan Liu, Joon T Kim, Amanda L Wiggenhorn, Julia T Tanzo, Alan Sheng-Hwa Tung, Xuchao Lyu, Peter-James H Zushin, Robert S Jansen, Basil Michael, Kang Yong Loh, Andrew C Yang, Christian S Carl, Christian T Voldstedlund, Wei Wei, Stephanie M Terrell, Benjamin C Moeller, Rick M Arthur, Gareth A Wallis, Koen van de Wetering, Andreas Stahl, Bente Kiens, Erik A Richter, Steven M Banik, Michael P Snyder, Yong Xu, Jonathan Z Long
Title: An exercise-inducible metabolite that suppresses feeding and obesity
by: Stanford University, Baylor College of Medicine, University of California Berkeley, Netherlands Cancer Institute, Radboud University, University of California San Francisco, University of Copenhagen, University of California at Davis, University of Birmingham, Thomas Jefferson University
Release Date: 2022-06-15
Website: Nature
Publisher: Springer Nature Limited

[s48] - https://bulletin.auburn.edu/coursesofinstruction/ansc/
Title: Auburn Bulletin 2024-2025
by: Auburn University
Release Date: 2024-2025
Website: Auburn University

[s49] - https://catalog.tamu.edu/graduate/course-descriptions/ansc/ansc.pdf
Title: ANSC - Animal Science
by: Texas A&M University
Website: Texas A&M University

[s50] - https://apps.ualberta.ca/catalogue/course/an_sc
Title: Animal Science Course Catalogue
by: University of Alberta
Website: ualberta.ca

[s51] - https://link.springer.com/article/10.1007/s12649-018-0351-5
Author: Izabela Michalak, Katarzyna Godlewska, Krzysztof Marycz
Title: Biomass Enriched with Minerals via Biosorption Process as a Potential Ingredient of Horse Feed
Release Date: 26 May 2018
Website: SpringerLink
Publisher: Springer

[s52] - https://www.equine74.com/blog/calcium-overdose-in-horses
Title: Calcium Overdose in Horses — by: Equine74
Website: Equine74

[s53] - https://madbarn.ca/feeds/mega-cell-mvp-pelleted-multi-vitamin-and-mineral-med-vet/
Title: Mega-Cell MVP – Pelleted Multi Vitamin and Mineral (Med-Vet) — by: Mad Barn
Website: Mad Barn

[s54] - https://madbarn.ca/feeds/phosphate-rock-soft/
Title: Phosphate – Rock Soft — by: Mad Barn
Website: Mad Barn

[s55] - https://www.agrobs.de/en/gipfelstuermer-mineral-p5106/
Title: Gipfelstürmer Mineral — by: AGROBS GmbH
Website: agrobs.de

[s56] - https://ceh.vetmed.ucdavis.edu/sites/g/files/dgvnsk4536/files/inline-files/Horse_Report_Fall_2018_web.pdf
Author: Carrie J. Finno, DVM, Ph.D. — Title: Horse Report
by: University of California, Davis — Release Date: Fall 2018
Website: Center for Equine Health — Publisher: University of California, Davis, School of Veterinary Medicine

[s57] - https://botupharma.com/download/mioprox02.pdf
Author: C.J. Finno and S.J. Valberg — Title: A Comparative Review of Vitamin E and Associated Equine Disorders
Release Date: 2012 — Website: botupharma.com
Publisher: American College of Veterinary Internal Medicine

[s58] - https://feedxl.com/vitamin-k-for-horses/
Author: FeedXL Equine Nutrition Team — Title: Vitamin K for Horses
by: FeedXL — Release Date: August 25, 2022
Website: FeedXL

[s59] - https://www.grandmeadows.com/the-science/vitamins-minerals/
Title: Vitamins & Minerals for Horses — by: Grand Meadows, Inc.
Website: Grand Meadows

[s60] - https://pubmed.ncbi.nlm.nih.gov/34331715/
Author: Erin N Hales, Hadi Habib, Gianna Favro, Scott Katzman, R Russell Sakai, Sabin Marquardt, Matthew H Bordbari, Brittni Ming-Whitfield, Janel Peterson, Anna R Dahlgren, Victor Rivas, Carolina Alanis Ramirez, Sichong Peng, Callum G Donnelly, Bobbi-Sue Dizmang, Angelica Kallenberg, Robert Grahn, Andrew D Miller, Kevin Woolard, Benjamin Moeller, Birgit Puschner, Carrie J Finno — Title: Increased α-tocopherol metabolism in horses with equine neuroaxonal dystrophy
by: University of California-Davis — Release Date: 2021-09
Website: PubMed — Publisher: Wiley Periodicals LLC on behalf of American College of Veterinary Internal Medicine

[s61] - https://pubmed.ncbi.nlm.nih.gov/16426221/
Author: Thomas J Divers, John E Cummings, Alexander de Lahunta, Harold F Hintz, Hussni O Mohammed — Title: Evaluation of the risk of motor neuron disease in horses fed a diet low in vitamin E and high in copper and iron
Release Date: 2006-01 — Website: PubMed
Publisher: American Journal of Veterinary Research

[s62] - https://www.distanceriding.org/wp-content/uploads/2017/09/Challenges-of-Endurance-Exercise-Hydration-and-Electrolyte-Depletion.pdf
Author: HAROLD C. SCHOTT II — Title: Challenges of Endurance Exercise: Hydration and Electrolyte Depletion
by: Michigan State University — Website: Distance Riding

[s63] - https://www.mdpi.com/2306-7381/9/11/626
Title: Evaluation of Resting Serum Bile Acid Concentrations in Dogs with Sepsis — by: MDPI
Website: MDPI

[s64] - https://training.arioneo.com/en/blog-thermoregulation-in-horses-how-does-he-regulate-his-body-heat/
Title: Thermoregulation in horses: how do they regulate their body heat? — by: Arioneo
Release Date: 2022-11-25 — Website: Arioneo Training

[s65] - https://animalsciences.rutgers.edu/faculty/mckeever/KennethMcKeever_Publications.pdf
Author: Kenneth H. McKeever, Ph.D., FACSM — Title: PUBLICATIONS
Website: Rutgers University — Publisher: Elsevier

[s66] - https://hyperdrug.co.uk/horse/supplements-for-horses/respiratory-supplements-for-horses/
Title: Respiratory Supplements for Horses — by: Hyperdrug
Website: hyperdrug.co.uk

[s67] - https://mrmjournal.biomedcentral.com/articles/10.1186/s40248-015-0010-7
Author: Charlotte Sandersen, Dorothee Bienzle, Simona Cerri, Thierry Franck, Sandrine Derochette, Philippe Neven, Ange Mouytis-Mickalad, Didier Serteyn — Title: Effect of inhaled hydrosoluble curcumin on inflammatory markers in broncho-alveolar lavage fluid of horses with LPS-induced lung neutrophilia
Release Date: 15 April 2015 — Website: Multidisciplinary Respiratory Medicine
Publisher: BMC

[s68] - https://real.mtak.hu/165540/1/Bartos_GALLEY.pdf
Author: Ádám Bartos, Nikoletta Such, Fruzsina Vanda Gál — Title: The effect of a fermented herbal feed supplement on the digestion of horses
by: Hungarian University of Agriculture and Life Science — Release Date: 2023
Website: Ecocycles — Publisher: European Ecocycles Society

[s69] - https://dengie.com/horse-feeds/healthy-range/healthy-tummy/
Title: Healthy Tummy — by: Dengie
Website: Dengie

[s70] - https://www.equinevitality.co.uk/
Title: Natural health supplements for horses and ponies — by: Equine Vitality
Website: Equine Vitality

[s71] - http://bmrat.org/index.php/BMRAT/article/view/685
Author: Niti Yashvardhini, Samiksha Samiksha, Deepak Kumar Jha — Title: Pharmacological intervention of various Indian medicinal plants in combating COVID-19 infection
Release Date: Jul 31, 2021 — Website: Biomedical Research and Therapy

[s72] - https://bmcvetres.biomedcentral.com/articles/10.1186/s12917-016-0714-8
Author: Hannah Ayrle, Meike Mevissen, Martin Kaske, Heiko Nathues, Niels Gruetzner, Matthias Melzig, Michael Walkenhorst
Title: Medicinal plants – prophylactic and therapeutic options for gastrointestinal and respiratory diseases in calves and piglets? A systematic review
by: BMC Veterinary Research
Release Date: 2016-06-06
Website: BMC Veterinary Research
Publisher: BioMed Central

[s73] - http://nanobioletters.com/wp-content/uploads/2022/10/LIANBS124.134.pdf
Author: Shobhit Prakash Srivastava, Saurav Yadav, Ratnesh Chaubey, Smriti Ojha, Ayush Chandra Mishra, Shalini Yadav, Sudhanshu Mishra
Title: Herbal Immunomodulators: A Powerful Preventive Weapon for COVID-19
by: Dr. M. C. Saxena College of Pharmacy, Lucknow, Uttar Pradesh, India; Department of Pharmaceutical Science & Technology Madan Mohan Malaviya University of Technology, Gorakhpur, Uttar Pradesh, India
Release Date: 25.09.2022
Website: nanobioletters.com

[s74] - https://www.happyathillhorsery.com/horse_wound_care_ISP_Relief.html
Title: Horse Wound Care and First Aid
by: Happyat Hill Horsery
Website: happyathillhorsery.com

[s75] - https://www.cfsph.iastate.edu/thelivestockproject/using-herbs-and-essential-oils-with-dr-karlene-stange-dvm/
Author: Dr. Karlene Stange, DVM
Title: Using herbs and essential oils with Dr. Karlene Stange DVM
by: The Livestock Project
Release Date: February 17, 2023
Website: Iowa State University

[s76] - https://www.sciencedaily.com/releases/2024/05/240502113715.htm
Author: Isabelle B. Laumer, Caroline Schuppli
Title: Wild orangutan treats wound with pain-relieving plant
by: Max-Planck-Gesellschaft
Release Date: 2024-05-02
Website: ScienceDaily
Publisher: Max-Planck-Gesellschaft

[s77] - https://www.ukvetequine.com/content/clinical/physiotherapy-for-neck-pain-in-the-horse/
Title: Physiotherapy for Neck Pain in the Horse
by: UK Vet Equine
Website: UK Vet Equine

[s78] - https://www.vetmed.auburn.edu/wp-content/uploads/2018/09/Overview-Of-Rehabilitation-Principles-.pdf
Author: Steve Adair MS, DVM, DACVS, DACVSMR
Title: Equine Rehabilitation
by: University of Tennessee Veterinary Medical Center
Website: Auburn University College of Veterinary Medicine

[s79] - https://equinemanualtherapist.com/
by: Equine Manual Therapist
Website: Equine Manual Therapist

[s80] - https://www.drbarbaraparks.com/career-certification-programs
Title: Career Certification Programs
by: Dr. Barbara Parks
Website: drbarbaraparks.com

[s81] - https://physioequinesolutions.com/2019/05/20/equine-rehabilitation/
Author: Dr. Emily Shields, PT, CCS, CERP
Title: Equine Rehabilitation
by: Physio Equine Solutions
Release Date: May 20, 2019
Website: Physio Equine Solutions

[s82] - https://www.resilientequine.com/blog/neurosomatic-therapy
Author: Jessica Parker
Title: NeuroSomatic Therapy
by: Resilient Equine
Release Date: Jul 10
Website: resilientequine.com

[s83] - https://vetmed.tennessee.edu/vmc/equinehospital/equineperformancerehab/
Title: Equine Performance & Rehabilitation
by: University of Tennessee
Website: University of Tennessee Veterinary Medical Center

[s84] - http://www.hendersonequineclinic.com/veterinary-kinesiotaping
Author: Dr. Bonny Henderson, Dr. Lauren Powell, Dr. Emily Tuttle
Title: Veterinary Kinesiotaping
by: Henderson Equine Clinic
Website: Henderson Equine Clinic

[s85] - https://www.jessicalimpkin.co.uk/jessica-limpkin-equine-massage-blog/kinesiology-taping-for-equine-therapists-with-jo-rose
Author: Jessica Limpkin
Title: Kinesiology Taping for Equine Therapists with Jo Rose
by: Rose Therapy
Release Date: November 19, 2021
Website: Jessica Limpkin Equine Massage Therapy

[s86] - https://www.ncsuvetce.com/product/equine-kinesiology-taping-course-ii-hands-on-lab-december-7th-2024-lake-worth-fl/
Title: Equine Kinesiology Taping Course II – (HANDS-ON LAB)
by: North Carolina State University
Release Date: December 7, 2024
Website: NCSU VetCE

[s87] - https://www.thysol.com.au/kinesiology-taping-courses/equine/
Title: Equine Kinesiology Taping Course
by: THYSOL
Website: thysol.com.au

[s88] - https://www.animantia.it/welfare-rehabilitation/equine-therapies/
Title: Equine Therapies
by: Animantia
Release Date: 2021-12-29
Website: animantia.it

[s89] - https://www.vetmed.auburn.edu/wp-content/uploads/2018/09/Overview-Of-Rehabilitation-Principles-.pdf
Author: Steve Adair MS, DVM, DACVS, DACVSMR
Title: Equine Rehabilitation
by: University of Tennessee Veterinary Medical Center
Website: Auburn University College of Veterinary Medicine

[s90] - https://www.theplaidhorse.com/2024/01/30/baby-steps-early-therapy-on-young-horses-will-pay-dividends-later/
Author: Laura Stephenson
Title: Baby Steps: Early Therapy On Young Horses Will Pay Dividends Later
by: The Plaid Horse
Release Date: 2024-01-30
Website: The Plaid Horse

[s91] - https://www.horsebarnsupplies.com/equine-rehabilitation
Title: 7 Physical Therapy Techniques Used to Reduce Chronic Pain in Horses
by: J&E Grill Manufacturing
Website: Horse Barn Supplies

[s92] - https://www.weitzequine.com/equine-acupuncture
Author: Dr. Melissa
Title: Equine Acupuncture
by: Weitz Equine Veterinary Services
Website: Weitz Equine

[s93] - https://www.midatlanticequine.com/integrative-medicine.html
Author: Dr. Sullivan
Title: Integrative Medicine
by: Mid-Atlantic Equine Medical Center
Website: Mid-Atlantic Equine Medical Center

[s94] - https://vetmed.tennessee.edu/vmc/equinehospital/equineacupuncture/
Title: Acupuncture and Chiropractic
Website: University of Tennessee College of Veterinary Medicine
by: University of Tennessee Institute of Agriculture

[s95] - https://www.research.va.gov/currents/0317-2.cfm
Author: Mitch Mirkin
by: U.S. Department of Veterans Affairs
Website: VA Research Currents
Title: Study: Electroacupuncture eases pain through stem-cell release
Release Date: March 16, 2017

[s96] - https://pubmed.ncbi.nlm.nih.gov/18550160/
Author: W A Schofield
by: Hagyard Equine Medical Institute
Website: PubMed
Title: Use of acupuncture in equine reproduction
Release Date: 2008-06-11
Publisher: Theriogenology

[s97] - https://pubmed.ncbi.nlm.nih.gov/15460072/
Author: D V Wilson, C E Berney, D L Peroni, D R Mullineaux, N E Robinson
by: Michigan State University
Website: PubMed
Title: The effects of a single acupuncture treatment in horses with severe recurrent airway obstruction
Release Date: 2004-09
Publisher: Equine Veterinary Journal

[s98] - https://bevas.eu/
Author: Dr. Emiel Van den Bosch
by: BEVAS (Belgian Veterinary Acupuncture Society)
Title: Veterinary Acupuncture Training and Certification
Website: bevas.eu

[s99] - https://veterinarypage.vetmed.ufl.edu/2018/10/15/new-uf-equine-acupuncture-center-opens-in-marion-county/
Author: Dr. Huisheng Xie
by: University of Florida
Website: veterinarypage.vetmed.ufl.edu
Title: New UF Equine Acupuncture Center opens in Marion County
Release Date: September 4, 2018
Publisher: University of Florida College of Veterinary Medicine

[s100] - https://www.equineosteopathy.org/
Title: Uniting the Profession of Equine Osteopathy
Website: Equine Osteopathy
by: Worldwide Alliance of Equine Osteopaths (WAEO)

[s101] - https://actavet.vfu.cz/media/pdf/actavet_2022091040347.pdf
Author: Giedrė Vokietytė -Vilėniškė, Simona Nagreckienė, Iveta Duliebaitė, Vytuolis Žilaitis
by: Lithuanian University of Health Sciences
Website: actavet.vfu.cz
Title: Effectiveness of cranial osteopathy therapy on nociception in equine back as evaluated by pressure algometry
Release Date: 2022-10-10
Publisher: ACTA VET. BRNO

[s102] - https://carolynmcgregorosteopath.com/carolyn-mcgregor-osteopathy-homoeopathy-healing/equine-and-animal-osteopathy-and-healing/
Author: Carolyn McGregor
Website: carolynmcgregorosteopath.com
Title: Equine and Animal Osteopathy with Healing

[s103] - https://international-animalhealth.com/wp-content/uploads/2017/12/Homeopathy-in-animals.pdf
Author: Peter Lees, Danny Chambers, Ludovic Pelligand, Pierre-Louis Toutain, Martin Whitehead
by: International Animal Health Journal
Title: Homeopathy in Animals: Yesterday and Today … But Tomorrow?
Website: International Animal Health

[s104] - https://pubmed.ncbi.nlm.nih.gov/11212087/
Author: M Elliott
by: Kingley Veterinary Centre
Website: PubMed
Title: Cushing's disease: a new approach to therapy in equine and canine patients
Release Date: 2001-01
Publisher: Br Homeopath J

[s105] - https://vetdergikafkas.org/uploads/pdf/pdf_KVFD_L_1974.pdf
Author: Çağla PARKAN YARAMIŞ, Marie-Noëlle ISSAUTIER, Sinem ULGEN SAKA, Berjan DEMIRTAŞ, Dilek OLGUN ERDIKMEN, Mehmet Erman OR
by: Istanbul University
Website: Kafkas University Veterinary Faculty Journal
Title: Homeopathic Treatments in 17 Horses with Stereotypic Behaviours
Release Date: 27.04.2016

[s106] - https://cam4animals.co.uk/veterinary-homeopathic-research/
Author: Dr. Petra Weiermayer
by: CAM4Animals
Website: CAM4Animals
Title: Veterinary homeopathic research
Release Date: 2019-04-18

[s107] - https://iavh.org/en/for-veterinarians/research/
Author: Dr. Petra Weiermayer
by: IAVH (International Association for Veterinary Homeopathy)
Title: Research in Veterinary Homeopathy
Website: IAVH

[s108] - https://www.nycavma.org/modalities.html
Title: Modalities
Website: NYCAVMA
by: New York Complementary & Alternative Veterinary Medical Association

[s109] - https://lakewoodanimalhospital.ca/wp-content/uploads/sites/106/2014/12/Bach-Flower-Remedies.pdf
Title: Bach Flower Remedies: Applications in Animals
Website: lakewoodanimalhospital.ca
by: Lakewood Animal Hospital

[s110] - http://www.hampshireholisticvet.co.uk/
Author: Dr. Dean Hawkins
by: Hampshire Veterinary Hospital
Title: Holistic Veterinary Medicine
Website: Hampshire Holistic Vet

[s111] - https://equinenaturalhealth.co.uk/rescue-remedy-for-horses/
Title: Rescue Remedy For Horses
Release Date: September 21, 2018
by: Equine Natural Health
Website: The Guide to Equine Natural Health

[s112] - https://www.bachfloweradvice.co.uk/bach-flowers-and-animals/bach-flower-for-horses
Author: Tom Vermeersch
by: Bach Flower Advice
Title: Bach Flower for Horses
Website: Bach Flower Advice

[s113] - https://www.creaturecomforters.org/flower-power.html
Author: Jane Stevenson
by: Creature Comforters
Website: Creature Comforters
Title: Flower Power! The natural way to ease stress
Release Date: June 2006

[s114] - https://www.blackdiamondvet.com/blog/evacuating-wildfires-with-horses
Author: Caelli Edmonds
by: Black Diamond Veterinary
Website: blackdiamondvet.com
Title: Evacuating Wildfires with Horses
Release Date: July 9, 2024

[s115] - https://www.aspcapro.org/resource/how-make-pet-first-aid-kit
Title: How to Make a Pet First Aid Kit
Website: ASPCApro
by: American Society for the Prevention of Cruelty to Animals (ASPCA)

[s116] - https://ddvh.com.au/management-of-equine-wounds-part-2-more-serious-wound-repair/

Author:	Darling Downs Vets	**Title:**	Management of equine wounds Part 2 – more serious wound repair
Release Date:	2017-11-23	**Website:**	Darling Downs Vets

[s117] - https://equineinstitute.org/new-blog/horse-first-aid-essentials

Author:	April Johnston	**Title:**	Horse First Aid Essentials: Be Prepared for Equine Emergencies on and off the Trail
by:	The Equine Institute	**Release Date:**	December 08, 2023
Website:	equineinstitute.org		

[s118] - https://equestrian.ca/wp-content/uploads/cdn/storage/resources_v2/Equine%20Care%20Program%20-%20Facility%20Manual%20EN%202022-08-11.pdf

Author:	Equestrian Canada	**Title:**	Equine Care Program - Facility Manual
Release Date:	2022-08-11	**Website:**	equestrian.ca

[s119] - https://vetmedbiosci.colostate.edu/vth/services/equine-field-service/equine-recommended-deworming-schedule/

Title:	Equine Recommended Deworming Schedule	**by:**	Colorado State University
Website:	Colorado State University Veterinary Teaching Hospital		

[s120] - https://ceh.vetmed.ucdavis.edu/sites/g/files/dgvnsk4536/files/local_resources/pdfs/pubs-July2013HR-sec.pdf

Author:	Dr. Claudia Sonder	**Title:**	Transporting Horses by Road and Air: Recommendations for Reducing the Stress
by:	Center for Equine Health	**Release Date:**	July 2013
Website:	University of California, Davis		

[s121] - https://www.fda.gov/animal-veterinary/animal-drug-compounding/qa-gfi-256-compounding-animal-drugs-bulk-drug-substances

Author:	U.S. Food and Drug Administration	**Title:**	Q&A: GFI #256 - Compounding Animal Drugs from Bulk Drug Substances
Release Date:	August 27, 2024	**Website:**	FDA

[s122] - https://aurorapharmaceutical.com/wp-content/uploads/2021/08/Essentials-V4-Iss-2-September-2021.pdf

Author:	Valerie Coerver, DVM	**Title:**	Essentials Volume 4 Issue 2
by:	Aurora Pharmaceutical, Inc.	**Release Date:**	September 2021
Website:	Aurora Pharmaceutical		

[s123] - https://www.cfsph.iastate.edu/Disinfection/Assets/Disinfection101.pdf

Title:	Disinfection 101	**by:**	CFSPH
Release Date:	2023	**Website:**	CFSPH

[s124] - https://pubmed.ncbi.nlm.nih.gov/7579639/

Author:	R M Dwyer	**Title:**	Disinfecting equine facilities
Release Date:	1995-06	**Website:**	PubMed
Publisher:	Rev Sci Tech		

[s125] - https://equine.ca.uky.edu/news-story/lots-elbow-grease-disinfection-project-0

Title:	Lots of Elbow Grease for Disinfection Project	**by:**	University of Kentucky
Release Date:	October, 2013	**Website:**	Ag Equine Programs

[s126] - https://www.cdfa.ca.gov/ahfss/animal_health/pdfs/I.pdf

Title:	Biosecurity- Keeping your Horse Healthy at Equine Events	**by:**	California Department of Food and Agriculture
Website:	California Department of Food and Agriculture		

[s127] - https://www.equineguelph.ca/pdf/facts/bio_security_info_FINAL.pdf

Author:	Alicia Skelding	**Title:**	Biosecurity for Horse Owners
by:	Equine Guelph	**Website:**	Equine Guelph
Publisher:	University of Guelph		

[s128] - https://www.vet.upenn.edu/about/news-room/bellwether/new-bolton-post/new-bolton-post-summer-2014/penn-vet-experts-advise-community-on-equine-herpes-virus

Author:	Louisa Shepard	**Title:**	Penn Vet Experts Advise Community on Equine Herpesvirus
by:	University of Pennsylvania School of Veterinary Medicine	**Release Date:**	Jul 21, 2014
Website:	University of Pennsylvania School of Veterinary Medicine		

[s129] - https://www.ed.ac.uk/sites/default/files/imports/fileManager/dvepfactsheet-woundcare.pdf

Title:	Dick Vet Equine Practice Fact Sheet: Wound Care	**by:**	Dick Vet Equine Practice
Website:	www.dickvetequine.com		

[s130] - https://www.vetvoice.com.au/ec/horses/wound-care/

Title:	Equine Wound Care	**by:**	Australian Veterinary Association
Website:	Vet Voice		

[s131] - https://blackdownequineclinic.com/wp-content/uploads/2017/12/Wounds_Fact_Sheet.pdf

Title:	Wound Care Fact Sheet	**by:**	Blackdown Equine Clinic
Website:	Blackdown Equine Clinic		

[s132] - https://ddvh.com.au/management-of-equine-wounds-part-1-what-horse-owners-need-to-know/

Author:	Darling Downs Vets	**Title:**	Management of equine wounds Part 1 – what horse owners need to know
Release Date:	2017-10-26	**Website:**	Darling Downs Vets
Publisher:	Horse Deals Magazine		

[s133] - https://vetmed.tamu.edu/news/pet-talk/topical-wound-care-for-horses/

Author:	Dr. Glennon Mays	**Title:**	Topical Wound Care for Horses
by:	Texas A&M University	**Release Date:**	June 2, 2011
Website:	Texas A&M College of Veterinary Medicine & Biomedical Sciences		

[s134] - https://alpineequine.net/blog/244653-novembers-focus-is-wound-healing-wound-management-in-the-horse-part-1

Title:	November's focus is wound healing-Wound Management in the horse-part 1	**by:**	Alpine Equine Hospital
Release Date:	Nov. 27, 2020	**Website:**	Alpine Equine

[s135] - https://www.liverpool.ac.uk/equine/common-conditions/colic/what-is-colic/

Title:	What is colic?	**by:**	University of Liverpool
Website:	University of Liverpool		

[s136] - https://www.ed.ac.uk/files/imports/fileManager/dvepfactsheet-colic.pdf

Title:	Colic Fact Sheet	**by:**	The Dick Vet Equine Practice
Website:	www.dickvetequine.com		

[s137] - https://vmc.usask.ca/care/equine-health/resources/colic.php

Title:	Equine Colic	**by:**	Western College of Veterinary Medicine
Website:	University of Saskatchewan		

[s138] - https://www.ivsajournals.com/article_157954_29f9421580f17dfd41c583917646fa4a.pdf

Author:	Seyed Mehdi Ghamsari, Fereidoon Saberi Afshar, Alireza Bashiri, Peyman Azizi, Omid Azari	**Title:**	Acute Equine Colic due to the Diaphragmatic Hernia: Two Cases
by:	Iranian Veterinary Surgery Association	**Release Date:**	24 September 2022
Website:	Iranian Journal of Veterinary Surgery		

[s139] - https://pubmed.ncbi.nlm.nih.gov/23428423/
Author: V E N Copas, A E Durham, C H Stratford, B C McGorum, B Waggett, R S Pirie **Title:** In equine grass sickness, serum amyloid A and fibrinogen are elevated, and can aid differential diagnosis from non-inflammatory causes of colic
by: Liphook Equine Hospital **Release Date:** 2013-04-13
Website: PubMed **Publisher:** Veterinary Record

[s140] - https://www.nj.gov/agriculture/animalemergency/prepare/disasteraction.shtml
Title: Disaster Action Guidelines for Horse and Livestock Owners **by:** New Jersey Department of Agriculture
Website: NJ.gov

[s141] - https://equineinstitute.org/new-blog/horse-injury-emergency-response
Author: April Johnston **Title:** Essential Horse Injury Emergency Response: Recognizing Signs, When to Call Vet, and Taking Action
by: The Equine Institute **Release Date:** December 01, 2023
Website: Equine Institute

[s142] - https://www.ksvhc.org/services/equine/timely-topics/trailtalk-june2023.html
Author: Dr. Bethany Roof **Title:** Equine Emergency Preparedness: Developing an Effective Equine Emergency Plan
by: Kansas State University **Release Date:** June 2023
Website: Kansas State University Veterinary Health Center

[s143] - https://equineinstitute.org/new-blog/heat-stroke-in-horses
Author: April Johnston **Title:** Quick Response to Heat Stroke in Horses: Effective First Aid Measures
by: The Equine Institute **Release Date:** December 01, 2023
Website: Equine Institute

[s144] - https://oldwaterlooequine.com/news-info/first-aid-kits/
Title: First Aid Kits **by:** Old Waterloo Equine Clinic
Website: oldwaterlooequine.com

[s145] - https://extension.colostate.edu/topic-areas/agriculture/wildfire-preparedness-for-horse-owners-1-817/
Author: N. Striegel **Title:** Wildfire Preparedness for Horse Owners – 1.817
by: Colorado State University Extension **Release Date:** 3/14
Website: Colorado State University Extension

[s146] - http://www.valleyequineveterinary.com/equine-services
by: Valley Equine Veterinary Service Inc **Website:** valleyequineveterinary.com

[s147] - https://www.eliteequinemobiledentistry.com/services
Title: Services **by:** Elite Equine Mobile Dentistry, PLLC
Website: Elite Equine Mobile Dentistry

[s148] - https://alpinehospital.com/healthy-teeth-happy-horse-2/
Author: Louise Marron, DVM **Title:** Healthy Teeth Happy Horse
by: Alpine Animal Hospital **Release Date:** Feb 2, 2017
Website: Alpine Animal Hospital

[s149] - https://alpineequine.net/dentistry-and-dental-surgery
Author: Dr. Maker **Title:** Dentistry and Dental Surgery
by: Alpine Equine Hospital **Website:** Alpine Equine

[s150] - https://www.evergreenequinevet.com/services/dentistry
Title: Dentistry **by:** Evergreen Equine Veterinary Practice
Release Date: 2024 **Website:** Evergreen Equine Veterinary Practice

[s151] - https://www.ksvhc.org/services/equine/timely-topics/trailtalk-April19-vaccinations.html
Title: Vaccination Reminders **by:** Kansas State University
Release Date: April 2019 **Website:** Kansas State University Veterinary Health Center

[s152] - https://leginfo.legislature.ca.gov/faces/codes_displaySection.xhtml?lawCode=BPC§ionNum=4827.
Title: Business and Professions Code - BPC Section 4827 **by:** California Legislature
Release Date: 2021-01-01 **Website:** leginfo.legislature.ca.gov

[s153] - https://www.depts.ttu.edu/vetschool/research/research-areas/disease-ecology-management-prevention-focus/index.php
Title: Faculty Disease Ecology, Management, and Prevention Research Focuses **by:** Texas Tech University
Website: Texas Tech University School of Veterinary Medicine

[s154] - https://vetmed.tamu.edu/dvm/resources/curriculum/
Title: DVM Professional Program Curriculum **by:** Texas A&M University
Website: Texas A&M College of Veterinary Medicine & Biomedical Sciences

[s155] - https://www.aspcapro.org/topics-shelter-medicine/intake-preventive-care
Title: Intake & Preventive Care **by:** American Society for the Prevention of Cruelty to Animals
Website: aspcapro.org

[s156] - https://vetmed.tennessee.edu/wp-content/uploads/sites/4/UTCVM_HorseParasiteControl.pdf
Author: Dr. Amy Lee Macintire & Dr. José R. Castro **Title:** Horse Parasite Control: Strategic Deworming
by: University of Tennessee College of Veterinary Medicine **Release Date:** 2018-12-21
Website: vetmed.tennessee.edu **Publisher:** University of Tennessee College of Veterinary Medicine

[s157] - https://vet.tufts.edu/tufts-veterinary-field-service/specialties-services/equine/routine-wellness-care
Title: Routine & Wellness Care **by:** Tufts Veterinary Field Service
Website: Tufts University

[s158] - https://vetmedbiosci.colostate.edu/vth/wp-content/uploads/sites/7/2021/01/recommended-equine-deworming-schedule.pdf
Title: Recommended Equine Deworming Schedule **by:** Colorado State University
Website: Colorado State University Veterinary Medicine and Biomedical Sciences

[s159] - https://vetmed.tamu.edu/news/pet-talk/texas-am-parasitologist-offers-suggestions-for-horse-deworming-treatments-in-texas/
Author: Dr. Thomas Craig **Title:** Texas A&M Parasitologist Offers Suggestions for Horse Deworming Treatments in Texas
by: Texas A&M University **Release Date:** July 20, 2012
Website: Texas A&M Veterinary Medicine & Biomedical Sciences

[s160] - https://edis.ifas.ufl.edu/publication/VM251
Author: Jennifer Bearden, Brittany Justesen, and Sally DeNotta **Title:** Developing a Deworming Program for Florida Horses
by: University of Florida **Release Date:** 2023-02-16
Website: UF/IFAS Extension **Publisher:** UF/IFAS Veterinary Medicine—Large Animal Clinical Sciences Department

[s161] - https://www.nwequinevet.com/services/vaccines-and-deworming
Title: Vaccinations and Deworming — by: Northwest Equine Veterinary Associates
Website: Northwest Equine Veterinary Associates

[s162] - https://aaep.org/wp-content/uploads/2024/05/Internal-Parasite-Guidelines_Updated.pdf
Author: AAEP — Title: AAEP Internal Parasite Control Guidelines
Release Date: 2024 — Website: aaep.org

[s163] - https://equineinstitute.org/new-blog/treating-hoof-ailments
Author: April Johnston — Title: Expert Tips for Treating Hoof Ailments & Boosting Horse Health
by: The Equine Institute — Release Date: December 01, 2023
Website: Equine Institute

[s164] - https://cavallofarms.com/equine-elegance-a-guide-to-happy-healthy-horse-care/
Title: Equine Elegance: A Guide to Happy & Healthy Horse Care — by: Cavallo Farms
Release Date: February 4, 2024 — Website: Cavallo Farms

[s165] - https://lifedatalabs.com/blog/tag/balanced-hooves/
Title: The Importance of Maintaining a Regular Farrier Schedule — by: Life Data Labs, Inc.
Release Date: March 30, 2018 — Website: Life Data® Blog

[s166] - https://reiterwelt.eu/blogs/our-latest-posts/why-do-horses-need-horseshoes
Title: Why do horses need horseshoes? — by: ReiterWelt
Release Date: May 10, 2024 — Website: ReiterWelt

[s167] - http://laneendfarm.com/farriery/
Title: Professional Farrier Services at Lane End Farm in Somerset — by: Lane End Farm
Website: Lane End Farm

[s168] - https://www.extension.purdue.edu/extmedia/id/id-321-w.pdf
Author: Kate Hepworth, Dr. Michael Neary, Dr. Simon Kenyon — Title: Hoof Anatomy, Care and Management in Livestock
by: Purdue University Cooperative Extension Service — Release Date: 10/04
Website: Purdue University Extension — Publisher: Purdue University Cooperative Extension Service

[s169] - https://www.lamenessprevention.org/site_page.cfm?pk_association_webpage_menu=6600
Title: E.L.P.O. Education Courses — by: Equine Lameness Prevention Organization
Website: Equine Lameness Prevention Organization

[s170] - https://www.nerdfitness.com/blog/how-to-build-your-own-workout-routine/
Author: Steve Kamb — Title: How To Build Your Own Workout Routine: Plans, Schedules, and Exercises
by: Nerd Fitness — Release Date: June 12, 2024
Website: Nerd Fitness

[s171] - https://research.med.psu.edu/oncology-nutrition-exercise/patient-guides/strength-training/
Title: Introduction to Strength Training — by: Penn State College of Medicine
Website: Penn State College of Medicine

[s172] - https://www.betterhealth.vic.gov.au/health/healthyliving/resistance-training-health-benefits
Title: Resistance training – health benefits — by: Better Health Channel
Release Date: 2007-07-31 — Website: Better Health Channel

[s173] - https://pubmed.ncbi.nlm.nih.gov/20847704/
Author: Brad J Schoenfeld — Title: The mechanisms of muscle hypertrophy and their application to resistance training
by: Global Fitness Services — Release Date: 2010-10
Website: PubMed — Publisher: J Strength Cond Res

[s174] - https://pubmed.ncbi.nlm.nih.gov/15064596/
Author: William J Kraemer, Nicholas A Ratamess — Title: Fundamentals of resistance training: progression and exercise prescription
Release Date: 2004-04 — Website: PubMed
Publisher: Med Sci Sports Exerc

[s175] - https://horsesport.com/magazine/health/developing-equine-athleticism-strength-fitness-plan/
Author: Jec Aristotle Ballou — Title: Developing Equine Athleticism: A Strength & Fitness Plan
by: Horse Sport — Release Date: June 10, 2024
Website: Horse Sport

[s176] - https://www.horsejournals.com/riding-training/english/dressage/best-cavalletti-exercises-walk-trot-and-canter
Author: Jec Aristotle Ballou — Title: The Best Cavalletti Exercises for Walk, Trot, and Canter
by: Canadian Horse Journal — Release Date: October 19, 2024
Website: Horse Journals

[s177] - https://www.horse-gym-2000.net/treadmill-study.html
Title: Treadmill Study — by: Horse Gym 2000 GmbH
Website: Horse Gym 2000

[s178] - https://christinakeim.com/2015/12/
Author: Christina Keim — Title: Motivating the Lazy Equine Athlete
Release Date: 2015-12-30 — Website: christinakeim.com

[s179] - https://www.distanceriding.org/condition-horse-like-pro/
Author: Nancy S. Loving, DVM — Title: Condition Your Horse Like a Pro
by: SEDRA (South Eastern Distance Riders Association) — Release Date: Apr 17, 2018
Website: distanceriding.org

[s180] - https://equestology.com.au/trainingscience/strengthtraining
Author: Equestology Sport Horse Science — Title: Strength Training For The Equine Athlete
Release Date: February 4, 2018 — Website: Equestology

[s181] - https://www.ukvetequine.com/content/clinical/muscle-hypertrophy-and-its-relevance-to-horses/
Title: Muscle Hypertrophy and Its Relevance to Horses — by: UK Vet Equine
Website: UK Vet Equine

[s182] - https://www.ukvetequine.com/content/clinical/muscle-hypertrophy-and-its-relevance-to-horses/
Title: Muscle Hypertrophy and Its Relevance to Horses — by: UK Vet Equine
Website: UK Vet Equine

[s183] - https://jps.biomedcentral.com/articles/10.1007/s12576-017-0575-3
Author: Hirofumi Miyata, Rika Itoh, Fumio Sato, Naoya Takebe, Tetsuro Hada, Teruaki Tozaki — Title: Effect of Myostatin SNP on muscle fiber properties in male Thoroughbred horses during training period
Release Date: 20 October 2017 — Website: The Journal of Physiological Sciences
Publisher: BMC

[s184] - https://rsdjournal.org/index.php/rsd/article/view/13204
Author: Paula Gomes Rodrigues, Katia de Oliveira, Stéphanie de Souza Vitório Alves, Camila Fernada Fidêncio, Clístenes Gomes de Oliveira, Lahesgyla Nascimento Fontes, José Miradelson Oliveira Carvalho, Camilla Mendonça Silva, Anselmo Domingos Ferreira Santos
by: Universidade Federal de Sergipe, Universidade Estadual Paulista
Title: Muscle and biomechanical response time in patrol horses submitted to functional training
Website: Research, Society and Development

[s185] - https://www.agrobs.de/en/know-how-advice/topics/building-muscle-through-diet-and-training-834/
Title: Building muscle through diet and training
Website: AGROBS
by: AGROBS GmbH

[s186] - https://nouvelleresearch.com/index.php/articles/14930-building-topline-horse-importance-of-nutrition-and-gut-health
Author: Tom Schell
by: Nouvelleresearch
Title: Building the Topline in the Horse; The Importance of Nutrition and Gut Health
Website: Nouvelleresearch

[s187] - https://www.vitafloor.com/news/tips-for-treating-soft-tissue-injuries-in-horses/
Title: Tips for Treating Soft Tissue Injuries in Horses
Release Date: 2023-08-11
by: Vitafloor
Website: Vitafloor

[s188] - https://www.mdpi.com/2076-2615/13/4/657
Title: Longitudinal Training and Workload Assessment in Young Friesian Stallions in Relation to Fitness, Part 2—An Adapted Training Program
Website: MDPI
by: MDPI
Publisher: MDPI

[s189] - https://vet.purdue.edu/esmc/files/documents/EHU%20Summer%202023.pdf
Author: Megan Bolger, DVM Class of 2023; Dr. Camilla Jamieson; Drs. Carla Olave and Emily Hess; Lindsey Takacs, DVM Class of 2023
by: Purdue University
Website: Purdue University College of Veterinary Medicine
Title: Equine Health Update
Release Date: 2023
Publisher: Donald J. McCrosky Equine Sports Medicine Center

[s190] - https://www.kohnkesown.com/wp-content/uploads/2020/07/C7-Sacroiliac-Pain-Factsheet-2020.pdf
Author: Dr John Kohnke BVSc RDA
by: Kohnke's Own
Website: Kohnke's Own
Title: Sacroiliac Pain
Release Date: 2020

[s191] - https://www.nature.com/articles/s41467-022-35390-3
Author: David E. Lee, Lauren K. McKay, Akshay Bareja, Yongwu Li, Alastair Khodabukus, Nenad Bursac, Gregory A. Taylor, Gurpreet S. Baht, James P. White
by: Nature Communications
Website: Nature
Title: Meteorin-like is an injectable peptide that can enhance regeneration in aged muscle through immune-driven fibro/adipogenic progenitor signaling
Release Date: 2022-12-09
Publisher: Nature Publishing Group

[s192] - https://veteriankey.com/biomechanics-of-locomotion-in-the-athletic-horse/
Author: Eric Barrey
by: Veterinary Key
Title: Biomechanics of locomotion in the athletic horse
Website: Veterinary Key

[s193] - https://pubmed.ncbi.nlm.nih.gov/6519042/
Author: D H Leach, K Ormrod, H M Clayton
Release Date: 1984-11
Publisher: Equine Veterinary Journal
Title: Standardised terminology for the description and analysis of equine locomotion
Website: PubMed

[s194] - https://edis.ifas.ufl.edu/publication/AN332
Author: Laura Patterson Rosa, Carissa Wickens, Samantha A. Brooks
by: University of Florida
Title: Genetic Selection for Gaits in the Horse
Website: UF/IFAS

[s195] - https://research.utwente.nl/files/299379592/Accurate_Horse_Gait.pdf
Author: Hamed Darbandi, Filipe Serra Bragança, Berend Jan van der Zwaag, Paul Havinga
by: University of Twente, Utrecht University
Website: University of Twente
Title: Accurate Horse Gait Event Estimation Using an Inertial Sensor Mounted on Different Body Locations
Release Date: 2022
Publisher: IEEE

[s196] - https://www.nature.com/articles/nature11399
Author: Lisa S. Andersson, Martin Larhammar, Fatima Memic, Hanna Wootz, Doreen Schwochow, Carl-Johan Rubin, Kalicharan Patra, Thorvaldur Arnason, Lisbeth Wellbring, Göran Hjälm, Freyja Imsland, Jessica L. Petersen, Molly E. McCue, James R. Mickelson, Gus Cothran, Nadav Ahituv, Lars Roepstorff, Sofia Mikko, Anna Vallstedt, Gabriella Lindgren, Leif Andersson, Klas Kullander
by: Nature
Website: nature.com
Title: Mutations in DMRT3 affect locomotion in horses and spinal circuit function in mice
Release Date: 29 August 2012

[s197] - https://www.nature.com/articles/s41467-024-47443-w
Author: Milad Shafiee, Guillaume Bellegarda, Auke Ijspeert
by: Nature Communications
Website: nature.com
Title: Viability leads to the emergence of gait transitions in learning agile quadrupedal locomotion on challenging terrains
Release Date: 09 April 2024
Publisher: Nature Publishing Group

[s198] - https://link.springer.com/article/10.1007/s10803-023-06174-5
Author: Juan Vives-Vilarroig, Paola Ruiz-Bernardo, Andrés García-Gómez
Release Date: 21 January 2024
Publisher: Journal of Autism and Developmental Disorders
Title: Effects of Horseback Riding on the Postural Control of Autistic Children: A Multiple Baseline Across-subjects Design
Website: Springer

[s199] - https://www.davethindmethod.com/blog/introspection-and-proprioception
Author: Dave Thind
by: Dave Thind Method
Website: Dave Thind Method
Title: Can Past Falls or Other Long-Ago Experiences Silently be Hindering Your Progress?
Release Date: 2023-09-29

[s200] - https://yourdressage.com/2019/10/09/the-neurologic-dressage-horse/
Author: Heather Smith Thomas
by: YourDressage.org
Website: YourDressage.org
Title: The Neurologic Dressage Horse
Release Date: 2019-10-09

[s201] - https://www.nature.com/articles/srep08169
Author: Yasuhiro Fukuoka, Yasushi Habu, Takahiro Fukui | Title: A simple rule for quadrupedal gait generation determined by leg loading feedback: a modeling study
by: Nature Publishing Group | Release Date: 2015-02-02
Website: Nature | Publisher: Scientific Reports

[s202] - https://www.horsejournals.com/riding-training/english/dressage/building-stronger-horses
Author: Jec A. Ballou | Title: Building Stronger Horses
by: Horse Journals | Release Date: October 4, 2020
Website: Horse Journals

[s203] - https://www.equitopiacenter.com/educators/dr-karin-liebbrandt/
Author: Dr. Karin Leibbrandt | Title: Horse Rehabilitation & Training
by: Equitopia Center | Website: Equitopia Center

[s204] - https://www.performancefooting.com/blog/horse-biomechanics/
Title: Horse Biomechanics: The Key to Optimal Performance | by: Performance Footing
Release Date: Aug 19, 2020 | Website: Performance Footing

[s205] - https://pubmed.ncbi.nlm.nih.gov/19406498/
Author: Miroslav Janura, Christian Peham, Tereza Dvorakova, Milan Elfmark | Title: An assessment of the pressure distribution exerted by a rider on the back of a horse during hippotherapy
by: Palacky University Olomouc | Release Date: 2009-04-29
Website: PubMed | Publisher: Hum Mov Sci

[s206] - https://jneuroengrehab.biomedcentral.com/articles/10.1186/s12984-021-00929-w
Author: Priscilla Lightsey, Yonghee Lee, Nancy Krenek, Pilwon Hur | Title: Physical therapy treatments incorporating equine movement: a pilot study exploring interactions between children with cerebral palsy and the horse
Release Date: 2021-09-06 | Website: Journal of NeuroEngineering and Rehabilitation
Publisher: BMC

[s207] - https://training.arioneo.com/en/the-racehorses-training-monitoring/
Author: Emmanuelle Van Erck | Title: Racehorse's Training Monitoring
by: Arioneo | Website: Arioneo

[s208] - https://www.alancouzens.com/blog/fitness_and_health.html
Author: Alan Couzens, MS (Sports Science) | Title: Fitness, Health and Performance: One but not the same. (Lessons from our horsey friends)
Release Date: March 14th, 2015 | Website: Alan Couzens

[s209] - https://www.e-jvc.org/journal/view.html?doi=10.17555/jvc.2023.40.6.464
Author: Seung-Ho Ryu, HeeEun Song, Eliot Forbes, Byung-Sun Kim, Joon-Gyu Kim, Ki-Jeong Na | Title: A Pilot Study on the Heart Rates of Jeju Horses during Race Trials
by: Korean Society of Veterinary Clinics | Release Date: December 31, 2023
Website: e-jvc.org

[s210] - https://hrvtraining.com/category/programming/
Author: Andrew Flatt Ph.D. | Title: Training Load and Nutrition Impact on HRV: 10 Week Data Analysis
by: HRVtraining | Release Date: 2013-12-06
Website: hrvtraining.com

[s211] - https://www.equinetendon.com/vitafloor-and-equine-tendon-announce-strategic-partnership-to-revolutionize-equine-rehabilitation/
Author: Scott Rawson | Title: Vitafloor and Equine Tendon Announce Strategic Partnership to Revolutionize Equine Rehabilitation
by: Vitafloor USA Inc. and Equine Tendon Ltd. | Release Date: August 13, 2024
Website: Equine Tendon

[s212] - https://bmcvetres.biomedcentral.com/articles/10.1186/s12917-017-0969-8
Author: Cornelis Marinus de Bruijn, Willem Houterman, Margreet Ploeg, Bart Ducro, Berit Boshuizen, Klaartje Goethals, Elisabeth-Lidwien Verdegaal, Catherine Delesalle | Title: Monitoring training response in young Friesian dressage horses using two different standardised exercise tests (SETs)
by: BMC Veterinary Research | Release Date: 14 February 2017
Website: BMC Veterinary Research | Publisher: BMC

[s213] - https://www.mdpi.com/2076-2615/13/4/689
Title: Putative Role of CFSH in the Eyestalk-AG-Testicular Endocrine Axis of the Swimming Crab Portunus trituberculatus | by: MDPI
Website: MDPI | Publisher: MDPI

[s214] - https://core.ac.uk/download/pdf/82145339.pdf
Author: Brad H. DeWeese, Guy Hornsby, Meg Stone, Michael H. Stone | Title: The training process: Planning for strength–power training in track and field. Part 2: Practical and applied aspects
by: Elsevier B.V. | Release Date: 17 July 2015
Website: ScienceDirect | Publisher: Shanghai University of Sport

[s215] - https://feelthebyrn.blog/tag/aging-athlete/
Author: Gordo Byrn | Title: Sunday Summary 20 November 2022
Release Date: November 20, 2022 | Website: Feel The Byrn

[s216] - https://en.magazine.clipmyhorse.tv/artikel/der-ultimative-leitfaden-zum-distanzreiten-alles-was-du-wissen-musst
Author: Sina Schulze | Title: Der ultimative Leitfaden zum Distanzreiten: Alles, was du wissen musst
by: ClipMyHorse.TV | Website: ClipMyHorse.TV

[s217] - https://www.sportsperformancebulletin.com/training/endurance-training/peaking-the-art-of-planning-and-tapering
Author: Andrew Hamilton | Title: Peaking: the art of planning and tapering
Website: Sports Performance Bulletin

[s218] - https://www.equineultrasound.com/educational-resources/prevention-of-tendon-and-ligament-injuries
Author: Dr. Carol Gillis DVM, PhD, DACVSMR | Title: Prevention of Tendon and Ligament Injuries
by: K9 Ultrasound | Release Date: Jan 19
Website: equineultrasound.com

[s219] - https://www.horsejournals.com/how/how-reduce-risk-training-related-injuries
Author: Jodie Santarossa, DVM, CVA, CERT | Title: How to Reduce the Risk of Training Related Injuries
by: Horse Journals | Release Date: October 11, 2024
Website: Horse Journals

[s220] - https://horsenetwork.com/2016/12/keeping-your-performance-horse-sound/
Author: Dr. David Ramey | Title: Keeping Your Performance Horse Sound
by: Horse Network | Release Date: December 10, 2016
Website: Horse Network

[s221] - https://vorl.vetmed.ucdavis.edu/sites/g/files/dgvnsk4731/files/inline-files/Racing_Injury_Prevention_Program_Report.pdf
Author:	Susan M. Stover, DVM, PhD, Dipl ACVS	**Title:**	Racing Injury Prevention Program Report
by:	University of California Davis	**Release Date:**	July 2011 - June 2013
Website:	University of California Davis	**Publisher:**	California Horse Racing Board

[s222] - https://vet.arioneo.com/en/blog/muscular-contractures-in-sport-horses-management-and-prevention-thanks-to-technology/
Title:	Muscular contractures in athletic horses: management and prevention through technology	**by:**	ARIONEO
Release Date:	May 31, 2023	**Website:**	vet.arioneo.com

Image Sources

Information about all following images
None of the images were modified, only the resolution was adjusted.
All images retain their original license.
Despite careful review, the accuracy and attribution of images cannot be guaranteed.
All images were finally retrieved and verified 2024-12-03.

Used Licenses

CC BY-SA 4.0	https://creativecommons.org/licenses/by-sa/4.0
No restrictions	https://www.flickr.com/commons/usage/
CC BY-SA 2.0	https://creativecommons.org/licenses/by-sa/2.0
CC BY 4.0	https://creativecommons.org/licenses/by/4.0
CC0	http://creativecommons.org/publicdomain/zero/1.0/deed.en
CC BY-SA 3.0	http://creativecommons.org/licenses/by-sa/3.0/
FAL	http://artlibre.org/licence/lal/en
GFDL 1.2	http://www.gnu.org/licenses/old-licenses/fdl-1.2.html
CC BY-SA 1.0	https://creativecommons.org/licenses/by-sa/1.0
CC BY-SA 3.0 de	https://creativecommons.org/licenses/by-sa/3.0/de/deed.en

Image Credits

[i1] - https://upload.wikimedia.org/wikipedia/commons/4/4a/Cartilage_hyaline1.jpg
Date: 2008-06-03 by: Echinaceapallida
License: CC BY-SA 4.0 (https://creativecommons.org/licenses/by-sa/4.0)

[i2] - https://upload.wikimedia.org/wikipedia/commons/1/1a/Renegade_Hoof_Boots_Classic.png
Date: 2022-06-09 by: Lwolfe63
License: CC BY-SA 4.0 (https://creativecommons.org/licenses/by-sa/4.0)

[i3] - https://upload.wikimedia.org/wikipedia/commons/e/ea/Sabot_en_babouche_01.jpg
Date: 2022-04-26 by: .Anja.
Artist: Anne Jea. License: CC BY-SA 4.0 (https://creativecommons.org/licenses/by-sa/4.0)

[i4] - https://upload.wikimedia.org/wikipedia/commons/7/7a/Veterinary_notes_for_horse_owners_-_a_manual_of_horse_medicine_and_surgery_%281903%29_%2814781823702%29.jpg
Date: 1903 by: Fæ
Artist: Internet Archive Book Images License: No restrictions (https://www.flickr.com/commons/usage/)

[i5] - https://upload.wikimedia.org/wikipedia/commons/f/f6/The_Horse_-_its_treatment_in_health_and_disease%2C_with_a_complete_guide_to_breeding%2C_training_and_management_%281905%29_%2814763801912%29.jpg
Date: 1905 by: Fæ
Artist: Internet Archive Book Images License: No restrictions (https://www.flickr.com/commons/usage/)

[i6] - https://upload.wikimedia.org/wikipedia/commons/9/91/Annual_report_of_the_American_Museum_of_Natural_History_for_the_year_%281907%29_%2818433410951%29_%28cropped%29.jpg
Date: 1907 by: Kersti Nebelsiek
Artist: Internet Archive Book Images License: No restrictions (https://www.flickr.com/commons/usage/)

[i7] - https://upload.wikimedia.org/wikipedia/commons/c/c0/Horse_nose_01.jpg
Date: 2023-07-21 by: .Anja.
Artist: Anja License: CC BY-SA 4.0 (https://creativecommons.org/licenses/by-sa/4.0)

[i8] - https://upload.wikimedia.org/wikipedia/commons/d/d5/Normal_lung_Alveoli_%283678762542%29.jpg
Date: 2008-07-10 by: Netha Hussain
Artist: Yale Rosen License: CC BY-SA 2.0 (https://creativecommons.org/licenses/by-sa/2.0)

[i9] - https://upload.wikimedia.org/wikipedia/commons/7/78/Purine_Nucleoside_Phosphorylase.jpg
Date: 2004-12-17 by: Chris 73
License: Public domain

[i10] - https://upload.wikimedia.org/wikipedia/commons/d/d2/Histological_Structure_of_Large_Intestine.jpg
Date: 2022-03-15 by: S.M.M.Musabbir Uddin
License: CC BY-SA 4.0 (https://creativecommons.org/licenses/by-sa/4.0)

[i11] - https://upload.wikimedia.org/wikipedia/commons/b/bc/E_coli_at_10000x%2C_original.jpg
Date: 2005-03 by: Brian0918
Artist: Photo byfkfkrErbe, digital colorization by License: Public domain
Christopher Pooley, both of USDA, ARS, EMU.

[i12] - https://upload.wikimedia.org/wikipedia/commons/c/c1/Horse_retinal_neuron.jpg
Date: 2021-03-26 by: Katshutko
License: CC BY 4.0 (https://creativecommons.org/licenses/by/4.0)

[i13] - https://upload.wikimedia.org/wikipedia/commons/8/89/Astrocyte.jpg
Date: 13 November 2005 by: File Upload Bot (Magnus Manske)
Artist: Lka License: Attribution

[i14] - https://upload.wikimedia.org/wikipedia/commons/7/77/Bovine_Pulmonary_Artery_Endothelial_Cells_Fluorescent_Image.jpg
Date: 2019-12-06 by: Erin Rod
License: CC BY 4.0 (https://creativecommons.org/licenses/by/4.0)

[i15] - https://upload.wikimedia.org/wikipedia/commons/d/db/Naturalis_Biodiversity_Center_-_Gypsum_-_mineral.jpg
Date: 2014-08-06 by: Hansmuller
Artist: Naturalis Biodiversity Center License: CC0 (http://creativecommons.org/publicdomain/zero/1.0/deed.en)

[i16] - https://upload.wikimedia.org/wikipedia/commons/4/40/Natural_Copper_Ore_Macro_1.JPG
Date: 2007-07-24 by: Digon3
License: CC BY-SA 3.0 (http://creativecommons.org/licenses/by-sa/3.0/)

[i17] - https://upload.wikimedia.org/wikipedia/commons/6/6a/Manganese_Ore.jpg
Date: 2015-03-20 by: Thamizhpparithi Maari
License: CC BY-SA 4.0 (https://creativecommons.org/licenses/by-sa/4.0)

[i18] - https://upload.wikimedia.org/wikipedia/commons/f/f9/Zinc_fragment_sublimed_and_1cm3_cube.jpg
Date: 2010-10-02 by: Alchemist-hp
License: FAL (http://artlibre.org/licence/lal/en)

[i19] - https://upload.wikimedia.org/wikipedia/commons/3/3d/Cholecalciferol-3d.png
Date: 5/6/07 by: Trlkly
Artist: Sbrools License: CC BY-SA 3.0 (http://creativecommons.org/licenses/by-sa/3.0/)

[i20] - https://upload.wikimedia.org/wikipedia/commons/d/d2/Cobalt_Sample.jpg
Date: 2014-11-30 by: Tjdenholm
Artist: Tim Denholm License: CC BY 4.0 (https://creativecommons.org/licenses/by/4.0)

[i21] - https://upload.wikimedia.org/wikipedia/commons/f/f0/Vitamin-E-from-xtal-3D-bs-17.png
Date: 2023-10-22 by: Benjah-bmm27
Artist: Ben Mills License: Public domain

[i22] - https://upload.wikimedia.org/wikipedia/commons/d/d9/Horse_drawn_hearse_horse_City_of_London_Cemetery_2_lighter.jpg
Date: 2020-04-23 by: Acabashi
License: CC BY-SA 4.0 (https://creativecommons.org/licenses/by-sa/4.0)

[i23] - https://upload.wikimedia.org/wikipedia/commons/e/ea/Thyme-Bundle.jpg
Date: 2011-09-28 by: Evan-Amos
License: CC0 (http://creativecommons.org/publicdomain/zero/1.0/deed.en)

[i24] - https://upload.wikimedia.org/wikipedia/commons/5/5b/Curcuma_longa_roots.jpg
Date: 2014-03-22 by: Laitche
Artist: Simon A. Eugster License: CC BY-SA 3.0 (https://creativecommons.org/licenses/by-sa/3.0)

[i25] - https://upload.wikimedia.org/wikipedia/commons/f/f3/Eucalyptus_trees_in_Agioi_Apostoli._Crete%2C_Greece.jpg
Date: 2019-09-13 by: Ввласенко
License: CC BY-SA 3.0 (https://creativecommons.org/licenses/by-sa/3.0)

[i26] - https://upload.wikimedia.org/wikipedia/commons/c/c0/Foeniculum_July_2011-1a.jpg
Date: 2011-07-07 by: Alvesgaspar
License: CC BY-SA 3.0 (https://creativecommons.org/licenses/by-sa/3.0)

[i27] - https://upload.wikimedia.org/wikipedia/commons/8/8c/Mentha_arvensis_-_p%C3%B5ldm%C3%BCnt_Keila.jpg
Date: 2013-07-11 by: Iifar
Artist: Ivar Leidus License: CC BY-SA 3.0 (https://creativecommons.org/licenses/by-sa/3.0)

[i28] - https://upload.wikimedia.org/wikipedia/commons/1/10/Salvia_pratensis_006.jpg
Date: 2012-06-16 by: Llez
Artist: H. Zell License: CC BY-SA 3.0 (https://creativecommons.org/licenses/by-sa/3.0)

[i29] - https://upload.wikimedia.org/wikipedia/commons/2/2f/Dried_Star_Anise_Fruit_Seeds.jpg
Date: 2017-11-12 by: Sanjay ach
Artist: Sanjay Acharya License: CC BY-SA 4.0 (https://creativecommons.org/licenses/by-sa/4.0)

[i30] - https://upload.wikimedia.org/wikipedia/commons/b/b5/Gesloten_bloem_van_de_paardenbloem_%28Taraxacum_officinale%29_09-05-2021._%28d.j.b%29_02.jpg
Date: 2021-05-09 by: Famberhorst
Artist: Dominicus Johannes Bergsma License: CC BY-SA 4.0 (https://creativecommons.org/licenses/by-sa/4.0)

[i31] - https://upload.wikimedia.org/wikipedia/commons/a/a7/Chamomile%40original_size.jpg
Date: 2005-05-28 by: Fir0002
License: GFDL 1.2 (http://www.gnu.org/licenses/old-licenses/fdl-1.2.html)

[i32] - https://upload.wikimedia.org/wikipedia/commons/7/78/Medicago_sativa_-_harilik_lutsern_Keilas.jpg
Date: 2013-07-25 by: Iifar
Artist: Ivar Leidus License: CC BY-SA 3.0 (https://creativecommons.org/licenses/by-sa/3.0)

[i33] - https://upload.wikimedia.org/wikipedia/commons/6/69/Echinacea_purpurea_in_Aboul.jpg
Date: 2017-07-17 by: Tournasol7
Artist: Krzysztof Golik License: CC BY-SA 4.0 (https://creativecommons.org/licenses/by-sa/4.0)

[i34] - https://upload.wikimedia.org/wikipedia/commons/b/be/00_0838_Frucht_der_Pflanze_%E2%80%9EEchtes_S%C3%BCssholz%E2%80%9C_%28Glycyrrhiza_glabra%29.jpg
Date: 2019-09-21   by: W. Bulach
License: CC BY-SA 4.0 (https://creativecommons.org/licenses/by-sa/4.0)

[i35] - https://upload.wikimedia.org/wikipedia/commons/1/14/Origanum_vulgare_-_harilik_pune.jpg
Date: 30 June 2013, 21:36:21   by: Iifar
Artist: Ivar Leidus   License: CC BY-SA 3.0 (https://creativecommons.org/licenses/by-sa/3.0)

[i36] - https://upload.wikimedia.org/wikipedia/commons/7/7e/Dry_Ginger_1.jpg
Date: 2018-09-06   by: Peiyushk
Artist: Piyush Kothari   License: CC BY-SA 4.0 (https://creativecommons.org/licenses/by-sa/4.0)

[i37] - https://upload.wikimedia.org/wikipedia/commons/b/b7/Knoblauch_%28Allium_sativum%29-20200621-RM-085344.jpg
Date: 2020-06-21   by: Ermell
License: CC BY-SA 4.0 (https://creativecommons.org/licenses/by-sa/4.0)

[i38] - https://upload.wikimedia.org/wikipedia/commons/d/dd/Moringa_oleifera_kz01.jpg
Date: 2024-02-21   by: Kenraiz
License: CC BY-SA 4.0 (https://creativecommons.org/licenses/by-sa/4.0)

[i39] - https://upload.wikimedia.org/wikipedia/commons/4/49/Plagiomnium_affine_laminazellen.jpeg
Date: created   by: René Esposito
Artist: Fabelfroh   License: CC BY-SA 3.0 (http://creativecommons.org/licenses/by-sa/3.0/)

[i40] - https://upload.wikimedia.org/wikipedia/commons/6/63/Calendula_officinalis_flowerbud_22122014_%281%29.jpg
Date: 2014-12-22   by: Joydeep
License: CC BY-SA 3.0 (https://creativecommons.org/licenses/by-sa/3.0)

[i41] - https://upload.wikimedia.org/wikipedia/commons/9/97/Hypericum_perforatum20110702_023.jpg
Date: 2011-07-02   by: Bff
License: CC BY-SA 4.0 (https://creativecommons.org/licenses/by-sa/4.0)

[i42] - https://upload.wikimedia.org/wikipedia/commons/3/37/Plantago_lanceolata_-_Kulna.jpg
Date: 20 June 2022, 22:02   by: Iifar
Artist: Ivar Leidus   License: CC BY-SA 4.0 (https://creativecommons.org/licenses/by-sa/4.0)

[i43] - https://upload.wikimedia.org/wikipedia/commons/9/94/Myrrh.JPG
Date: 14 February 2005   by: Gaius Cornelius
License: Public domain

[i44] - https://upload.wikimedia.org/wikipedia/commons/4/4c/Dr.Umasankar_Mohanty_Demonstrating_Manual_Therapy_Techniques.jpg
Date: 2009-01-18   by: Prof.mohanty
License: CC BY-SA 4.0 (https://creativecommons.org/licenses/by-sa/4.0)

[i45] - https://upload.wikimedia.org/wikipedia/commons/2/24/KT_tape_on_the_back_of_adult_male.jpg
Date: 2021-02-27   by: Whoisjohngalt
License: CC BY-SA 4.0 (https://creativecommons.org/licenses/by-sa/4.0)

[i46] - https://upload.wikimedia.org/wikipedia/commons/7/77/Shiatsu_massage_set-up.jpg
Date: 2007-10-08   by: Flickr upload bot
Artist: Lee Haywood   License: CC BY-SA 2.0 (https://creativecommons.org/licenses/by-sa/2.0)

[i47] - https://upload.wikimedia.org/wikipedia/commons/3/30/Ost%C3%A9opathie_%C3%A9quine_ESOAA.JPG
Date: 2008-09-08   by: Animatum
License: CC BY-SA 3.0 (https://creativecommons.org/licenses/by-sa/3.0)

[i48] - https://upload.wikimedia.org/wikipedia/commons/5/58/Mare_repro_palpate_%285877979030%29.jpg
Date: 2008-04-08   by: Montanabw
Artist: eXtensionHorses   License: CC BY-SA 2.0 (https://creativecommons.org/licenses/by-sa/2.0)

[i49] - https://upload.wikimedia.org/wikipedia/commons/c/c3/Homeopathic_Medicine.jpg
Date: 2020-10-05   by: Dr. Moumita Sahana
License: CC BY-SA 4.0 (https://creativecommons.org/licenses/by-sa/4.0)

[i50] - https://upload.wikimedia.org/wikipedia/commons/8/8f/Grooming_Horse_by_Robert_Polhill_Bevan_-_Robert_Polhill_Bevan_-_ABDAG002290.jpg
Date: 1909   by: Watty62
Artist: class="fn value"> Robert Polhill Bevan   License: Public domain

[i51] - https://upload.wikimedia.org/wikipedia/commons/f/f6/Kuskokwim_Reconnaissance_expedition_members_leading_horses_across_ice_field_on_the_west_side_of_Simpson_Pass%2C_Alaska_Range_%28AL%2BCA_3763%29.jpg
Date: August   by: BMacZeroBot
Artist: class="fn value"> Unknown author   License: Public domain

[i52] - https://upload.wikimedia.org/wikipedia/commons/f/fa/Zaniskari_Horse_in_Ladakh.jpg
Date: 2018-06-26   by: Justlettersandnumbers
Artist: Eatcha   License: CC BY-SA 4.0 (https://creativecommons.org/licenses/by-sa/4.0)

[i53] - https://upload.wikimedia.org/wikipedia/commons/5/52/BMW_Polo_Masters_Meg%C3%A8ve_2014_-_bandages.jpg
Date: 2014-01-26   by: Ludo29
Artist: Ludovic Péron   License: CC BY-SA 3.0 (https://creativecommons.org/licenses/by-sa/3.0)

[i54] - https://upload.wikimedia.org/wikipedia/commons/8/80/Self-adhering-bandage.png
Date: 2020-03-23   by: Baedr-9439
License: CC0 (http://creativecommons.org/publicdomain/zero/1.0/deed.en)

[i55] - https://upload.wikimedia.org/wikipedia/commons/f/f7/Rotavirus.jpg
Date: 2006-01-24   by: Ciszewski W~commonswiki
Artist: F.P. Williams, U.S. EPA   License: Public domain

[i56] - https://upload.wikimedia.org/wikipedia/commons/b/b7/Human_fibrinogen_3GHG.png
Date: 2019-11-14   by: 5-HT2AR
License: CC0 (http://creativecommons.org/publicdomain/zero/1.0/deed.en)

[i57] - https://upload.wikimedia.org/wikipedia/commons/2/26/160504-A-PY568-001_%2826328283963%29.jpg
Date: 2016-05-10   by: Vanished Account Byeznhpyxeuztibuo
Artist: U.S. Department of Defense Current Photos   License: Public domain

[i58] - https://upload.wikimedia.org/wikipedia/commons/0/03/Horse-Vaccination.jpeg
Date: 1940   by: Eubulides
Artist: United States. Farm Security Administration.   License: Public domain
Office of War Information Photograph Collection.
Photographer is Wilbur Staats.

[i59] - https://upload.wikimedia.org/wikipedia/commons/c/c5/A_blacksmith_at_work.jpg
Date: 2009-08-24   by: Wizard191
Artist: Moose Jaw Times Herald   License: CC BY-SA 1.0
(https://creativecommons.org/licenses/by-sa/1.0)

[i60] - https://upload.wikimedia.org/wikipedia/commons/a/af/Hooves_with_special_horseshoes_02.jpg
Date: 2024-08-11   by: Kritzolina
License: CC BY-SA 4.0
(https://creativecommons.org/licenses/by-sa/4.0)

[i61] - https://upload.wikimedia.org/wikipedia/commons/9/9b/Chestnut_horse_hoof.JPG
Date: 2014-04-29   by: Montanabw
License: CC BY-SA 3.0
(https://creativecommons.org/licenses/by-sa/3.0)

[i62] - https://upload.wikimedia.org/wikipedia/commons/a/ac/Man_jumping_over_a_pommel_horse._Man_waiting_in_line_behin
d_him%2C_NINO_F_Scholten_photographic_print_19_1449.tiff
Date: Between   by: Mr.Nostalgic
Artist: Frank Scholten   License: Public domain

[i63] - https://upload.wikimedia.org/wikipedia/commons/8/86/Cavaletti_Systembalken_aus_verletzungsfreiem_Kunststoff.jpg
Date: 2016-10-01   by: Wdwdbot
Artist: Sylvia Naundorf   License: CC BY-SA 3.0 de
(https://creativecommons.org/licenses/by-sa/3.0/de/deed.en)

[i64] - https://upload.wikimedia.org/wikipedia/commons/4/4e/Horse_Altai_05.jpg
Date: 2013-06-08   by: Alexandr frolov
License: CC BY-SA 4.0
(https://creativecommons.org/licenses/by-sa/4.0)

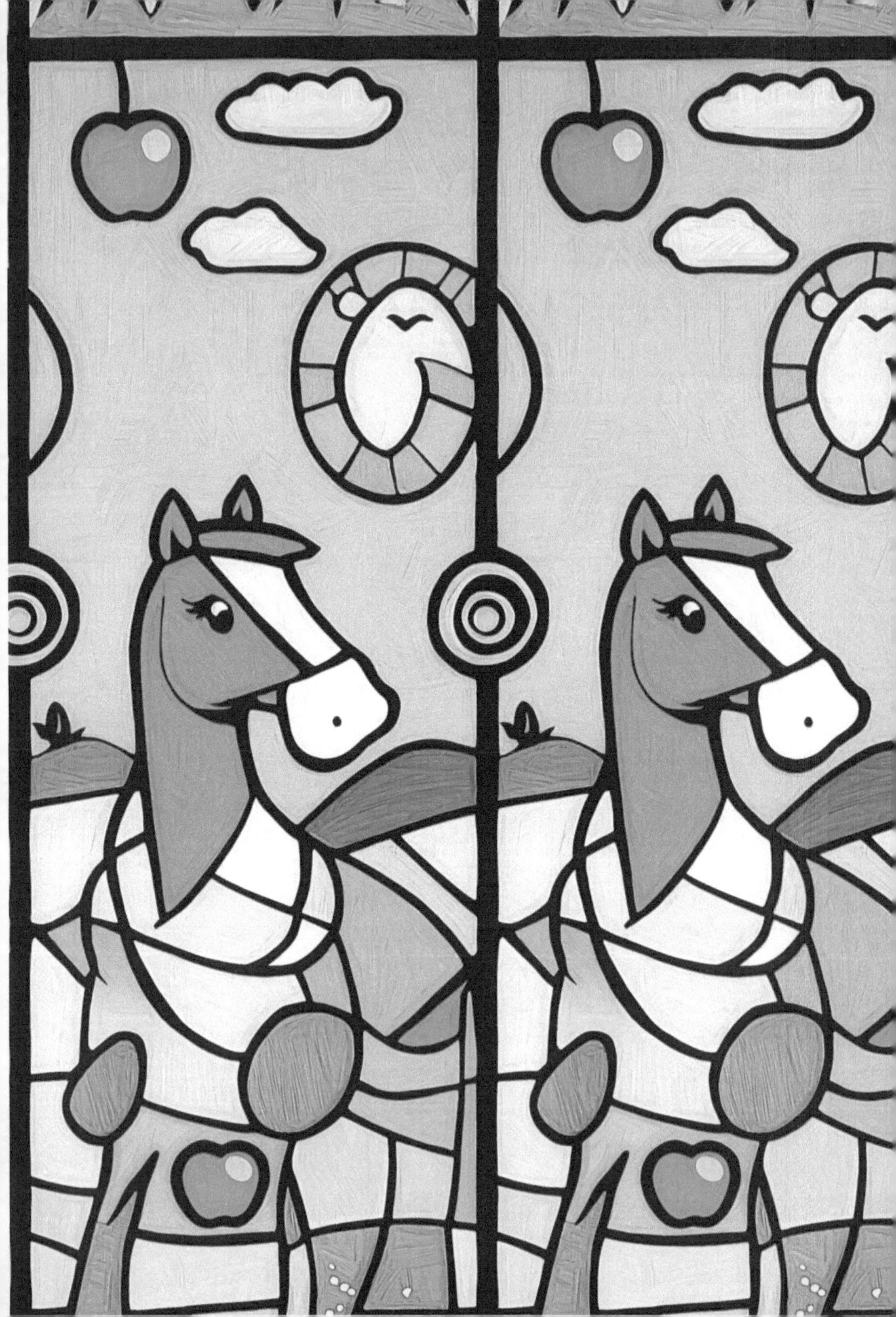